Juice Cleanse Solution

A Simple 7 Day Weight Loss Plan To Rid Stubborn Body Fat, Feel Energetic and Detox Without It Feeling Like One

Kathryn Young

By reading this document, the reader agrees that under no circumstances is the author responsible for any losses, direct or indirect, that are incurred as a result of the use of the information contained within this document, including, but not limited to, errors, omissions, or inaccuracies.

Special Bonus

Get the Bonus Report that includes:

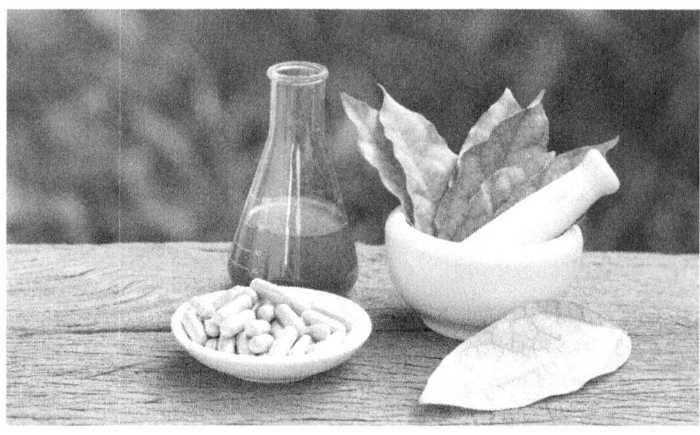

- ☐ Weight loss supplement buying guide
- ☐ Why **MOST** diets fail
- ☐ Alternative medicine tricks that worked for me

Get it now, visit the link:

bit.ly/healthybonus

TABLE OF CONTENTS

Introduction

"It is health that is the real wealth and not pieces of gold and silver."

- Mahatma Gandhi

Do you feel tired all the time? Does it feel like your weight loss has hit a wall, and you aren't able to lose fat? Regardless of how hard you exercise, are you finding it difficult to lose weight? Do you want to improve your overall health and body metabolism? If yes, then perhaps a detox is what your body needs. Following a juice cleanse is the perfect detox your body needs while improving your energy levels and meeting your weight loss goals.

I am sure you have heard of various detoxes and cleanses. One such detox is a juice cleanse. This book is the perfect guide for you to learn everything about a juice cleanse. Even better, you can attain all the benefits of a juice cleanse without feeling like you are following a restrictive diet. You will mostly be drinking your way to a healthier and fitter body.

A juice cleanse, as the name suggests, is a simple detox diet wherein you will be consuming plenty of fruit and vegetable juices. You no longer have to cook elaborate meals to follow this simple diet. All the juices you consume will provide your body with the nutrients and minerals it needs. Forget about spending hours together in the kitchen; all it takes is a couple of minutes to whip up a juice equivalent to an entire meal. So, even if you have a hectic schedule, you can easily follow this diet. This diet not only works but is incredibly easy to follow. A juice cleanse improves your metabolism, gives your body plenty of nutrition, helps internal detoxification, improves your energy levels, and much more. By following this simple diet for just a week, you can see an improvement in your overall health and well-being. A simple detox is all your body needs to start functioning optimally.

In this book, you will learn about a juice cleanse and signs your body needs to detoxify itself, different myths associated with a juice cleanse, and the various benefits it offers. You will also learn about how to start a juice cleanse, how it helps with weight loss, FAQs about a juice cleanse, tips to start a juice cleanse, and maintenance tips for after the cleanse. Apart from this, there are various juicing recipes given in this book you can use while following this diet.

The key to your good health lies in your hands, so take action today! Are you eager to learn more about all of this? If yes, then let us get started without further ado!

Chapter One:

The Secret to Success - How A Juice Cleanse Works

Signs You Need a Detox

We are surrounded by toxins, from the air we breathe to the water we drink and the food we eat. Toxins are present everywhere. These toxins tend to accumulate within your body, and once they reach their breaking point, they can make you ill. I have collated a few symptoms that may be passed off as regular daily issues, but they can lead to major problems if they persist. If you notice any of the symptoms discussed in this section, it is a sign your body needs a detox.

Brain Fog

Even after getting a good night's sleep, if you feel foggy, dizzy, lethargic, or have a tough time concentrating, it could be the result of toxins present within. These toxins tend to react severely with essential minerals and vitamins that your body requires to function optimally. This reaction is quite similar to something that would happen when you use the wrong fuel to power your car.

Constipation

We are inadvertently feeding our body plenty of chemicals like colorants, artificial flavorings, and preservatives whenever we consume processed foods. The digestive system helps digest all the food, but it also has to deal with the toxins. When these toxins are not removed from the body, they start building up and can cause digestive troubles like constipation. Consuming organic food, increasing your water intake, and avoiding alcohol can help resolve this issue.

Difficulty Sleeping

The buildup of harmful toxins in the body can make you feel exhausted, and to make things worse, it spoils your sleep routine. The presence of high levels of toxins disrupt the functioning of cortisol, a sleep-controlling hormone. Therefore, the buildup of toxins negatively affects your sleep cycle. Insomnia, when left unchecked, can cause other illnesses. Therefore, if you notice any difficulty falling and staying asleep, it could be a sign that your body desperately needs a detox.

Body Odor

Your body is not only regularly exposed to toxins but has to deal with the toxins that are present within it. So, your body starts to digest them, which leads to the production of foul-smelling gasses and odors. When these odors escape through your skin, it leads to body odor. Regardless of how often you shower or the deodorants you use, this odor will not go away. If you notice this, it is time for a body detox.

Body Aches

Even if you haven't been exercising vigorously or don't engage in any physically tiring activities, you might notice joint pains and muscle pains. A primary reason for this could be toxin buildup. Any form of unidentifiable body pain or ache is usually an indicator of unchecked inflammation in the body. If you cannot find any other apparent cause for inflammation, it could be a sign your body needs a detox.

Weight Gain

You are probably working out quite regularly and exercising, but notice that you are gaining weight or have stopped losing weight. Perhaps it could be something associated with the impact of hormones in your body. Toxins tend to harm certain hormones that regulate and maintain your weight. By following a healthy and organic diet routine like a juice cleanse, you can detoxify your body from within.

Skin Blemishes

The largest organ in the body that is continuously exposed to all sorts of pollution and pollutants is your skin. Certain body products like soaps, shampoos, lotions, or conditioners can contain harmful chemicals. When your digestive system doesn't function optimally because of the overload of toxins, it affects the health of your skin. Your skin helps eliminate toxins that are in your body. When your internal mechanism is compromised, it presents itself as various skin problems like acne, eczema, and rashes. When all this is combined with the harmful chemicals found in skincare products, it only worsens skin blemishes.

Brittle Nails

The toxins present in your body are pulled down due to gravitational force, and it directly affects your toenails. If you wear shoes all day long, then your toes stay within the confines of socks and shoes, creating the perfect ecosystem for fungus. Toxins, when coupled with this ecosystem, make your toenails quite attractive for fungal growths. If you notice that your toenails start looking brittle or ugly, it is a sign of toxin overload.

Bad Breath

Bad breath is usually a symptom associated with digestive troubles. When your digestive system is struggling to thoroughly digest and process all the food you consume, it can cause bad breath. However, if your liver is struggling to cleanse all the toxins present, it can cause digestive problems. The only way to tackle this problem is by detoxifying your body.

Hair Loss

Hair loss is a common symptom of toxic overload within the body. It could be caused because of harmful toxins like lead, arsenic, or thallium (present in cigarette smoke), among other toxins, which can make you severely sick. Therefore, never treat hair loss lightly.

Pay close attention to the way your body feels, and whenever you notice any of these symptoms, it is time for a detox.

About Juice Cleanses

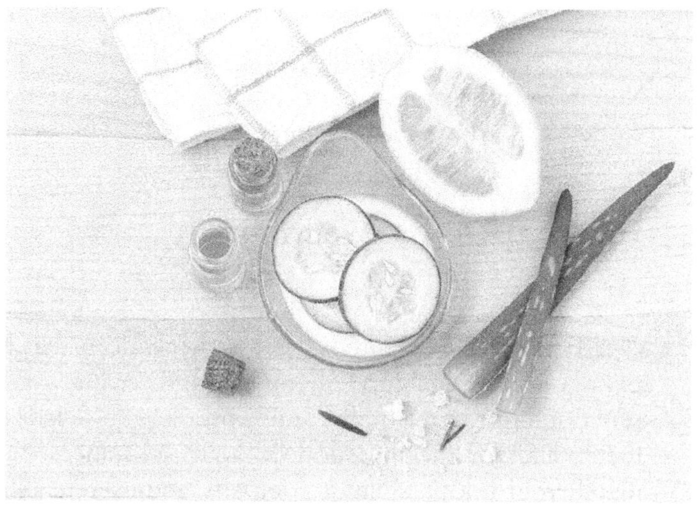

A juice cleanse is a detox diet wherein you will mainly be consuming vegetable and fruit juices for anywhere between 1 to 7 days. It is also known as a juice fast. There are a variety of juice cleanses, and some involve consumption of homemade juices, while others allow the consumption of store-bought juices.

The idea of making juices from fresh fruits, vegetables, and herbs for the different health benefits associated with them is not a new concept. Somewhere in the 1930s, the first modern juicing machine was invented. Since then, alternative health practitioners have recommended juicing as a means to tackle various ailments. Vegetable and fruit juices are filled with various nutrients and minerals. Juicing helps effectively extract all these nutrients and makes it easier for the body to digest and absorb them. Drinking healthy juices helps flush out toxins and toxic waste while filling it with helpful nutrients. A juice cleanse helps support your body's internal detox mechanism. Since this diet is usually devoid of caffeine, sugar, and other refined foods, it promotes a healthy way of eating.

You will learn more about a juice cleanse and how it works in the subsequent chapters.

Internal Detox Mechanism

Our bodies have an internal detox mechanism that helps fight off the buildup of toxins and ensure optimal functioning. If your body cannot produce sufficient toxic metabolites or the ingestion of toxic substances doesn't match your body's ability to detoxify and excrete all of it, it starts storing them within connective tissues. This, in turn, prevents them from concentrating on important tasks like defense and regulation. Detoxification essentially helps restore your body's regulatory mechanisms and enables the internal processes to start functioning normally. The different organs in the body, which help with detoxification are the liver, kidneys, respiratory tract, skin, and the intestines.

The Liver

The liver not only helps with digestion and regulation of hormones, but it also enables the proper functioning of your entire body. It is believed to be the body's primary center for detoxification. It helps deactivate and remove all sorts of toxic substances present within the food you consume like harmful minerals, excess hormones, food additives, or even toxic medications. It helps extract all the residual wastes present in the blood and transforms them so they can be easily removed by the kidneys or intestine. It also gets rid of the waste products, and all toxic metabolites produced because of intestinal fermentation or putrefaction.

The Kidneys

Kidneys help purify the blood and remove any harmful substances like chemicals and other toxic medications. It essentially filters them out of the blood and removes them from the body in the form of urine. The renal filters get clogged because of a high concentration of toxins in the blood, especially the chemical or synthetic substances that are not a part of the regular biological cycle. The filtration system in kidneys will not function optimally unless you start regulating the food you consume.

The Intestines

The intestinal tract extends from the mouth to the colon. It not only helps with digestion but also eliminates toxins. After the food goes through different phases of digestion, the different nutrients present in it, like fats, sugars, vitamins, minerals, amino acids, etc., are transported to the liver for redistribution. After detoxifying all this, the liver redistributes these helpful nutrients to different parts of the body. During this process, the undesirable chemicals or toxins are dumped into the bile by the liver. Bile helps transport all this to the small intestine, and then it is processed through the intestinal tract until removed as excreta. When there is a toxin overload, all the toxins stay within the intestinal tract and are not converted into fecal matter. After a while, they tend to putrefy and ferment, causing a variety of digestive troubles.

The Skin

If the liver, kidneys, and intestines don't perform the tasks optimally, your body depends on the skin for removing toxins. Skin is the largest organ present in the body, and it not only acts as a protective and defensive mechanism, but it is a sensory organ, too. The skin eliminates most of the toxins present within in the form of sweat. When the food you consume is rich in refined sugars or is quite acidic, other types of residual wastes and toxins are removed by the skin in the form of rashes or pimples.

If there is an excessive buildup of toxins within your

body, then these systems cannot function optimally. Following a detoxification diet like the juice cleanse helps optimize their ability to detoxify your body from within.

How a Juice Cleanse Works

During a juice cleanse, you will be required to consume only fruit or vegetable juices for the duration of the cleanse. A regular juice cleanse divided into three crucial stages.

Stage 1: Preparation

The first stage is all about preparing your body for the cleanse. It is also known as a pre-cleanse. 1 to 7 days before the juice cleanse, you must slowly eliminate certain foods like refined sugars, coffee, dairy products, meat, nicotine, and alcohol from your daily diet. By removing these foods, any withdrawal symptoms associated with shifting to a new diet like headaches, tiredness, fluctuations in energy levels, or cravings can be avoided. Or, if not prevented, the intensity can be considerably reduced. During this stage, you must start increasing your intake of fruits, vegetables, and fluids. Also, make a conscious decision to add a couple of fruit and vegetable juices to your daily diet. It makes it easier for your body to get used to the juice cleanse.

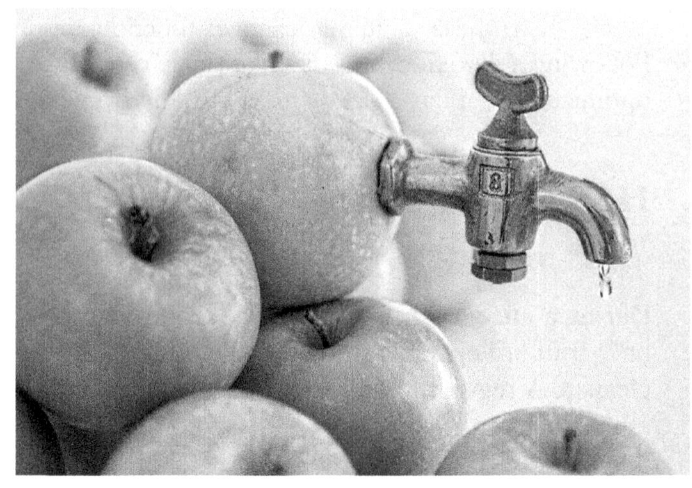

Stage 2: The Cleanse

A juice cleanse can last for anywhere between 1 to 7 days This is the actual cleanse, and during this period, you must consume at least 2 liters of fresh vegetable and fruit juices daily. At least half of the juice you consume must be from vegetables.

Stage 3: After the Cleanse

Once the cleanse is over, you must slowly ease your body back into your usual diet. Start by gradually reintroducing the foods you eliminated during the first stage. This stage can take up to 5 days.

You will learn in detail about all three stages in subsequent chapters.

Myths About Juice Cleanses

Juice cleanses are steadily gaining popularity because of all the different benefits they offer. In this section, let us look at some of the myths and facts about a juice cleanse.

Myth #1: No fiber

It is a common misconception that there is no fiber present in juices. Well, there are two types of fiber, and they are known as soluble and insoluble fiber. Juice contains plenty of soluble fibers. Whenever you juice fruits or vegetables, most of the insoluble fiber is removed after juicing, while the soluble fiber stays. Soluble fiber is like a sponge and offers bulking matter. It primarily supports the growth of good bacteria and promotes digestive health, since it acts like a prebiotic. So, you don't have to worry about not giving your body sufficient fiber while following the juice cleanse.

Myth #2: Juice detoxes don't work

A juice cleanse helps detoxify your body. That said, your body has an internal detox mechanism, and at times because of the buildup of toxins, this mechanism doesn't function as optimally as it is supposed to. If you follow a juice cleanse, it helps improve your body's ability to detox itself. For instance, the consumption of cruciferous vegetables like brussels sprouts, broccoli, cauliflower, radish, cabbage, and kale helps increase the production of liver enzymes, which help in detoxification. By adding these beneficial ingredients to your regular juicing routine, you improve your body's internal detoxification system.

Myth #3: There are no health benefits

Another popular misconception about juice cleanses is that they offer no health benefits whatsoever. With increasing research about the benefits of a well-balanced, plant-based diet, the benefits of juice cleanse are coming to light. For example, drinking juice made of beetroots helps reduce blood pressure levels. It has plenty of nitric oxide present in it, which improves your overall endurance while exercising. Another obvious benefit of a juice cleanse is that it helps detoxify your body by promoting the expulsion of toxins. You will learn more about the different health benefits of a juice cleanse in the subsequent sections.

Myth #4: Too much sugar

All juices are not created equally. If you follow the 80:20

(vegetables: fruits) ratio, then you don't have to worry about increasing your sugar intake. Even if certain fruits feel a little sugary, they offer plenty of health benefits. For instance, most berries are quite sweet, but they are rich in vitamins, antioxidants, and low in carbs. So, as long as you stick to a balanced intake of fruits and vegetables, your sugar levels will stay stabilized.

Myth #5: No protein

A classic criticism about a juice cleanse is that it doesn't provide the body with sufficient protein. If you are worried about your protein intake while following a juice cleanse, you can always add healthy protein supplements like hemp seeds, chia seeds, or even plant-based protein powders. For a healthy adult, there won't be any serious deficiency of protein even if you stick to a juice cleanse for a couple of days. By ensuring that you are consuming healthy and wholesome ingredients in the form of juices, you will not deprive your body of the protein it requires to function optimally.

Myth #6: Loss of nutrients

Another common misconception about juicing is that most of the nutrients are lost whenever the pulp is extracted. Well, you might lose a couple of nutrients like magnesium and fiber present in the pulp. However, you do provide your body with various other nutrients present in the juice. So, loss of nutrients is a minimal side effect, and it can easily be compensated for. Follow the simple juicing recipes given in this book, and you can ensure that all your nutritional requirements are met.

Myth #7: It is a fad

A juice cleanse might sound like a fad diet, but it certainly isn't. The benefits of juicing have been used by mankind since time immemorial. Juicing is not a new concept, and it has been around for ages now. There is plenty of research being conducted, and most of the results derived from it are positive. For instance, it is believed that carrot juice can help reverse the damage caused to white blood cell DNA in smokers.

Myth #8: Eating fruits and vegetables is better

Another popular misconception is that eating vegetables and fruits is much better than juicing. Well, in the end, all that matters is the intake of plant-based foods. As long as the destination stays the same, the vehicle used to get there doesn't matter. Regardless of whether it is in the form of a salad or a healthy juice if you are consuming the required amount of fruits and vegetables, your body gets all the nutrients it needs. So, you don't have to worry about harming your body and can start a juice cleanse today. Ensure that you consume a variety of fruits and vegetables to get the entire spectrum of nutrients your body needs.

Myth #9: It's expensive

A juice cleanse doesn't have to be expensive, and you don't necessarily need to splurge on costly ingredients. Juicing is not wasteful, and all the pulp you obtain can be reused. You can use it to make soups, burger patties, cookies, bread, crackers, and so much more. This diet is restrictive only if you believe it to be. So, don't hold yourself back and try to experiment as much as you can. If you want to reduce the costs involved, try to include as much seasonal produce as you probably can. You can also use frozen fruit to reduce the overall costs. Make the juices at home, and it will further reduce the costs. Bottled and packed juices often contain additives and other ingredients, which will do your body no good. They offer convenience, but that is the only benefit.

Myth #10: High risk of contamination

The risk of contamination is high only when juices are not made and stored properly. Instead of purchasing premade bottled juices, start making everything at home. To do this, you can follow the simple recipes given in this book. When you start making the juices at home, you have complete control over the ingredients you use, the quantity produced, and the kitchen environment. Clean all the equipment before you start using it. Most of the material used in facilities for mass-producing foods or juices are usually the source of contamination. Before you begin juicing any ingredients, don't forget to peel them. Peels often contain traces of pesticides and chemicals. Also, don't store these juices for prolonged periods, try to consume them immediately.

Replacing the myths with facts will undoubtedly ease your mind of any worries you have about a juice cleanse. Whenever something starts gaining popularity, plenty of myths start popping up about it. Learning to differentiate fact from fiction enables you to get a better understanding of the topic.

All the toxins that keep getting accumulated within your body tend to make you feel foggy and sluggish. It can also harm your overall health while affecting your sleep schedule. A juice cleanse is an incredibly simple protocol for cleansing your body from within. It not only provides the minerals and vitamins your body requires to get through the day, but by consuming liquid foods, you give your body a much-deserved break from sugar, fat, and various other pollutants. A juice cleanse effectively flushes out any environmental and dietary toxins present within your body while improving your immune system and assisting in weight loss.

Chapter Two:

A Quick Path to Weight Loss - How A Juice Cleanse Can Help

Overall Calorie Intake

Pretty much anything and everything you consume has certain calories present within. Except for a few calorie-free beverages like water, unsweetened black coffee, and unsweetened green or herbal teas, calories are present in everything else. If weight loss is your priority, then you must pay attention to the calories you consume. Your body must be in a state of a calorie deficit for weight loss. A calorie deficit occurs only when your calorie intake is less than your body's calorie expenditure. You don't necessarily have to cut down on the food you consume to maintain a calorie deficit. Instead, it is all about making healthy and wholesome choices.

People usually opt for a juice cleanse, since they want to

detoxify their body or speed up the process of weight loss. If these two things sound like your primary goals, then you must certainly pay attention to the calories you consume. Here is a necessary explanation of all the different calories present in fruit or vegetable juices. Fruit juices have higher calorie content since they are rich in carbs. On the other hand, vegetable juices are full of vitamins and nutrients instead of carbohydrates and therefore contain fewer calories. To maintain your overall health, it is vital that there is a sufficient balance between nutrients and minerals you consume while ensuring that your body gets enough calories to function optimally. Therefore, you must combine fruit and vegetable juices.

While following a juice cleanse, if you start depriving your body of the minimum calories it requires, it does more harm than good. You will not lose weight by starving your body. Instead, you must pay attention to the sources of calories you feed your body. Starvation is never equal to weight loss. So, let go of this misconception that drastically reducing your calorie intake is helpful for weight loss.

While following the basic juice cleanse, your daily intake of juices might be anywhere between 4 to 5 glasses. It virtually means you'll be consuming about 1.5 to 2 liters of fruit and vegetable juices daily. It is believed that one liter of juice can contain anywhere between 300 to 600 calories according to the ingredients you use. So, on the juice cleanse, your ideal intake of calories will be restricted to 900 to 1200 calories. Your daily calorie intake will depend on your body's needs. Never starve your body of the essential calories it needs to function optimally. Once your body is in starvation mode, it stops digesting the food or burning fats and starts diverting all the energy towards primary body functions required for survival. This, in turn, will halt any weight loss. The ideal calorie intake for an average adult is between 1600 to 2500 calories. While following a juice cleanse, your overall calorie intake will be reduced to half, even if that is not what you are trying to do. This, in turn, will effectively shift your body into a calorie deficit. Once your body is in a calorie deficit, it promotes weight loss.

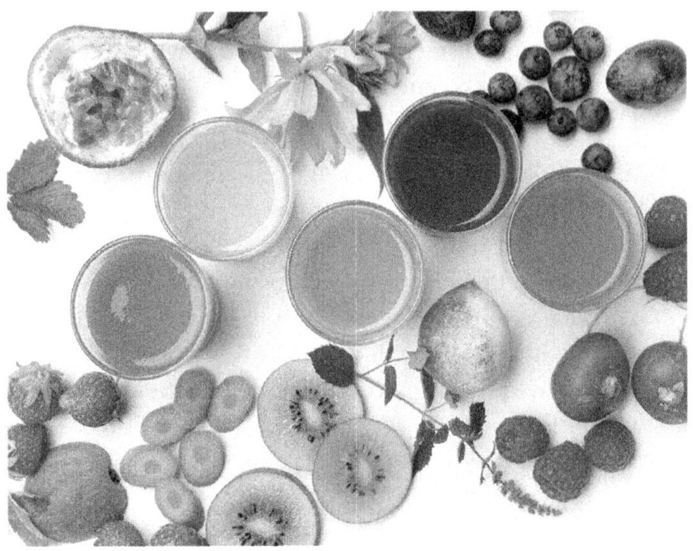

The total calories present in any juice primarily depends on the ingredients you decide to use. However, calculating your daily calorie intake is quite simple. Fruit juices tend to contain between 30 to 60 calories for 100 grams. So, if your daily intake of fruit juice is about 1 liter, your body will consume anywhere between 300 to 600 calories. Vegetable juices, on the other hand, especially green leafy vegetable juices, contain fewer calories.

Approximately 1 liter of any green vegetable juice can hold between 200 to 400 calories. So, if you consume 1 liter of vegetable juice, your body gets 200 to 400 calories. All in all, combining one liter of fruit and vegetable juices will give your body 500 to 1000 calories for two liters of juice you drink. 2 liters of fluids might not sound like much, but they are positively filling because of all the soluble fiber they contain.

Counting calories can become tricky since there are a variety of ingredients. In this section, let us look at some of the basic calorie estimates present in 100 grams of fruits and vegetables.

- Strawberries - 24 calories
- Watermelon - 29 calories
- Pomegranate - 66 calories
- Apple - 48 calories
- Cherries - 54 calories
- Blueberry - 47 calories
- Plum - 39 calories
- Banana - 78 calories
- Orange - 38 calories
- Grapes - 45 calories
- Guava - 45 calories
- Kiwi - 49 calories
- Papaya - 36 calories
- Pear - 54 calories
- Mango - 54 calories
- Kale - 34 calories
- Spinach - 14 calories

- Cucumber - 14 calories
- Cabbage - 15 calories
- Broccoli - 23 calories
- Beetroot - 32 calories
- Carrots - 30 calories
- Tomatoes - 13 calories
- Parsley - 36 calories
- Swiss chard -19 calories
- Wheatgrass - 21 calories
- Celery - 14 calories

Note: Keep in mind that these are rough estimates. If weight loss is your priority, then paying attention to your daily calorie intake is a good idea. Keep this list handy to calculate your daily calorie intake. When coupled with a little exercise, you can effectively and efficiently speed up the process of weight loss.

Juice Cleanse and Energy Levels

Juices certainly give your body a much-deserved energy boost. A juice cleanse not only improves your overall physical performance but also provides your brain with all the helpful nutrients it requires for optimal functioning. You will naturally feel more energetic when your body gets all the vitamins and nutrients it needs at regular intervals. If you are used to consuming coffee or any other energy drinks to feel energetic, then replace them with healthy juices. Instead of reaching for a cup of coffee, try replacing it with a healthy juice made of green leafy vegetables to feel energetic. Start your day on a refreshing note with a glass of vegetable or fruit juice, and you will not feel tired or sluggish. If you are running low on energy or feel like you don't have the required energy to get through a day, opt for a juice cleanse.

When there is an excessive buildup of toxins, and your body cannot move them effectively, it can make you feel exhausted and sluggish. Therefore, a juice cleanse will certainly help reverse the situation. Another factor that plays a vital role in your overall energy levels is the quality of sleep you manage to get. If your body doesn't get the sufficient sleep it requires or if you get disturbed sleep, then you will end up feeling tired and sluggish in the morning. When your body doesn't get the rest it needs to recharge its batteries, you cannot feel energetic.

Now, it is time to look at your usual lifestyle. If your regular lifestyle is predominantly sedentary, it is time to start adding some form of exercise to your usual routine.

A sedentary lifestyle can also reduce your overall energy levels and make you feel sluggish. Also, if you want to enter a state of calorie deficit, then your calorie expenditure must increase. The simplest way to do this is by adding exercise to your routine. Your diet also plays a significant role in your overall energy levels. A diet rich in sugars, carbs, and other processed foods will make you feel tired and sluggish. To effectively correct and reverse all these situations, a juice cleanse will come in handy.

If you're looking for a quick boost of energy, then here are a couple of things you must never forget. For a quick boost of energy, add plenty of leafy greens to your juices. Add parsley to the juice to improve your overall energy levels. Instead of increasing your intake of fruit juices, try to increase your intake of vegetable juices. Not only are vegetable juices low in calories, but the nutrients present in them can effectively clear your mind and give you plenty of energy. Try to add wheatgrass to the juices you consume. Even if it isn't the tastiest of juices, it is refreshing and energizing.

One final factor you must pay attention to is your caffeine intake. Consuming excessive caffeine might make you feel momentarily energetic, but when you experience a caffeine crash, you will feel sluggish and tired. To avoid this, limit your caffeine intake, and don't consume any caffeine late in the day. Excessive intake of caffeine also harms your sleeping schedule. If you are unable to fall asleep at night or stay asleep, then avoid consuming caffeine late in the day. In fact, while following the juice cleanse, try avoiding caffeine altogether, and you will feel more energetic.

Juice Cleanse and Metabolism

If you are interested in attaining your weight loss or fitness goals while improving your overall wellbeing, then a juice cleanse will come in handy. As stated in the previous section, there are a variety of benefits associated with juicing. In fact, you can start consuming fresh juices to kickstart your day instead of a cup of coffee. If you are used to drinking coffee early in the morning, then it will take your body a while to get used to this change. However, once your body gets used to it, you will never want to go back to your previous routine. Also, you will start to feel incredibly better about yourself, knowing that you are giving your body all the nutrients and vitamins it requires to function optimally. After all, you are the only one who can regulate and control your health. If you are not mindful of the food you feed your body, it will adversely affect your overall health.

The healing power of juices is quite incredible. Whenever you consume fresh juices made of vegetables and fruits, you are giving your body the essential fuel for functioning optimally. Not only juices are healthy, but they are tasty and help revitalize your body while restoring your overall vitality. Juicing certainly offers some healing powers, but how does it boost your metabolism? A quick Google search might tell you that the healing power of juicing is because of all the nutrients, minerals, and antioxidants present in the ingredients that supercharge your body. This might make you wonder why you are supposed to juice these ingredients when you can eat them? Well, the healing properties of the juice cleanse are based on two underlying factors. The first factor is associated with the various raw nutrients present, and the second factor is how they help in digestion and assimilation of the nutrients. Now, let's learn more about these two factors.

Fruits and vegetables are healthy for your body. This is not a secret, and no one would refute it. Fruits and vegetables also promote natural healing. However, it is always better to consume them in their raw form, instead of cooking them. Whenever food is cooked, certain nutrients present in them are effectively destroyed, since they are exposed to heat. Cooking is essentially a chemical process at a molecular level, which transforms the structure of different molecules in the ingredients. Therefore, the end product becomes a little foreign to your body. If you still have your doubts about this, ask yourself a simple question. What will happen if you place your hand in a pan of boiling water? How will your hand feel once it is exposed to such high degrees of heat? Do you think your hand would feel better, or would you be hurt? Well, obviously, you will end up burning your hand. Likewise, whenever you start cooking certain raw ingredients, the helpful enzymes present in them are destroyed. Now, what are these enzymes?

A lot of people forget that enzymes are as crucial as minerals, fats, carbs, proteins, water, and vitamins. If the food you consume doesn't have any enzymes present in it, you are essentially forcing your body to start expending its supply of proteins. All processed foods are devoid of the essential natural enzymes. Enzymes are the life force required for maintaining your optimal health and overall wellbeing. So, if you consume processed food, prepackaged food, or anything else that looks like it was mass-produced in a factory, your body must dip into its internal supply of enzymes to compensate for the absence of enzymes in the food consumed.

When the food you eat is exposed to external heat, the nutrients present in it are either wholly or partially destroyed. In a sense, the nutrients are denatured, and then, in turn, become toxic for your body. So, when it comes to consuming raw or cooked vegetables and fruits, it is always better to consume them in the raw and natural form. Juicing helps preserve and maintain the integrity of all the raw nutrients in the ingredients while effectively converting them into an easily and readily digestible form.

Several digestive processes and changes take place within your body because of juicing. Whenever you consume any food, your body automatically digests it. During digestion, your body absorbs all the various nutrients and minerals present in the food. Whatever is left over is assimilated and then subsequently removed. Your digestive system enables your body to attain this objective. The food you consume is immediately transformed into fuel required to carry out essential functions.

So, why is it essential that you must be mindful of your diet? Well, the food you consume provides your body with the nutrients it needs, and therefore, determines your overall well being. A simple fact a lot of people seem to ignore is that the human digestive system is not biologically designed for digesting certain foods. The list of foods your body has a tough time digesting include processed foods, refined foods, red meats, and dairy products. There is an ongoing debate in the fitness community about the benefits and drawbacks of consuming meat and dairy. In the last couple of decades, several dietary changes have been made to the essential human diet. So, biology is still trying to catch up with all these nutritional changes. Natural evolution has yet not caught up. The concept of healthy eating is slowly disappearing with the introduction of various processed foods. The consumption of denatured food tends to clog up your internal systems and prevents them from functioning optimally. This, in turn, means your digestive system cannot perform its functions as effectively and efficiently as it is intended to.

All these reasons, when put together, prove why juicing is a wonderful idea. Whenever you choose raw fruits and vegetables, you are reducing your body's work. The digestive system is almost like your body's natural juicer. When you consume solid food, this internal juicer is put to work to digest and absorb all that you consume. When you drink juices, you have simplified the digestive process altogether. Apart from that, you are also providing the vital raw nutrients for energizing your bodily functions. Juicing is a healthy and delicious method filled with fresh nutrients your body requires. Keep in mind that digestion is a process that requires some energy. About 10% of all the energy your body produces from the food you consume is shifted towards digestive purposes. If your body needs more energy to digest all that you eat, the remainder of energy will not be that much. To efficiently reverse this process, start juicing today.

A juice cleanse not only helps detoxify your body, but it also assists in weight loss. While following the juice cleanse, your overall calorie intake reduces, even if you don't pay any conscious attention to it. Apart from that, it also optimizes your level of hydration while eliminating unnecessary processed foods associated with weight gain. This, in turn, effectively helps kickstart the weight loss process. If you want to maintain the weight loss, it is essential that you make a couple of dietary and lifestyle changes once the cleanse ends.

Chapter Three:

The Magic of Detox- What A Juice Cleanse Can Do for Your Body

Modern life is all about convenience. We have not only come up with various inventions to make our lives easier, but these days, even food has become all about convenience. Walk into any grocery store, and you will be surrounded by different prepackaged and ready to eat options. When everything is this simple, is it any wonder health problems are increasing by the day? Well, the convenience that we all hold so dearly is the reason for it all. Convenience makes our life easy, but it harms our health in the long run. Not only are most of these prepackaged foods unhealthy, but they are devoid of nutritional value too. The romance with unhealthy foods is steadily increasing and is the root cause of several health problems plaguing humanity.

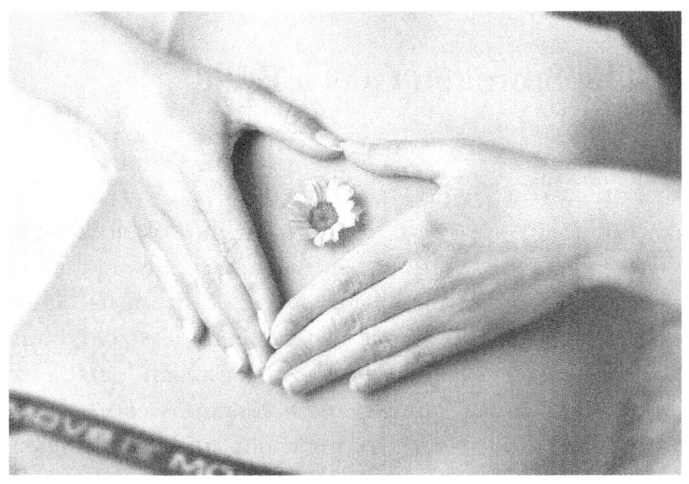

Unhealthy foods are not just the reason for obesity and weight gain, but for a variety of health conditions ranging from inflammation to cardiovascular dysfunctions. Therefore, it is important that you break free of this cycle of terrible dependence on refined carbs, processed sugars, saturated fats, and excessive caffeine or alcohol. The simplest way to reverse all this is by merely changing your diet. Yes, by making your diet plant-based instead of processed food-based, you can quickly turn your health around. By following the juice cleanse, you can not only break free of this vicious cycle of dependence on unhealthy foods, but you can also improve your overall health. In this section, let us look at the different ways in which a juice cleanse can help your body and health.

The Stomach Gets a Break

For anyone who takes medication to suppress the production of acid in the stomach and for all those whose stomachs don't produce sufficient acid, giving it a break is a good idea. Drinking juices reduce the usual strain the stomach is under. Since juices require less acid, churning, and pepsin for digestion, the stomach gets a much-deserved break from its usual functions. To further ease the metabolism, try to mindfully and slowly chew the juices to add some oral enzymes to it. How do you feel after working for long hours? You will feel tired. Now, how would you feel after getting some rest after a tiring day? You will feel refreshed and relaxed. Likewise, a juice cleanse works along these lines by giving your stomach a break and re-energizing it.

Gives the Liver a Break

It is not just the stomach that needs a break; even your liver needs a break from time to time. The liver is the primary center for detoxification. All the molecules absorbed from food tend to pass through the intestinal wall (except fiber), and then they are moved to the liver for detoxification. They are thoroughly detoxified and prepared before they are allowed to enter the other cells in the body. When there is an excessive buildup of toxins in the liver, or if the liver is overworked, most of these molecules pass unchecked and enter the general system of circulation. From there, they then move onto all the cells in the body and can wreak havoc. Following the simple organic juice cleanse helps relieve the overload on the liver and gives it a reprieve from its usual functions.

Improves the Gut's Health

Refined carbs, food additives, saturated fats, and pesticides are present in the food you consume, and other allergens, are all toxic to the gut. When these toxic foods are combined with medication like antacids or antibiotics, it further increases the stress on the gut. All this added stress can effectively impair your intestines and their ability to function optimally. It can also lead to an imbalance in the gut microbiome while resulting in many tears in the intestinal walls. The thin lining of the intestines prevents undigested food from entering the bloodstream. When this membrane is harmed due to toxic foods, it results in a condition known as leaky gut. Leaky gut essentially means unprocessed food molecules leak into the bloodstream. Consuming a diet that's rich in plant-based ingredients allows quick assimilation through the intestines. This process doesn't consume as much energy as the digestion of regular food. Therefore, a toxin-free and nutrient-dense diet like a juice cleanse helps improve your gut's health. When your gut starts functioning correctly, it improves your overall health.

Reduction in Appetite

Most of us are used to snacking constantly, and it usually is junk food. When you start eliminating all these foods from your diet and replace them with healthy juices, you overall appetite reduces. Juicing helps get rid of the habi of comfort eating, and enables your body to feel full, even when your food intake reduces. This kind of physiologica boost comes in handy, especially while making any dietary changes. Also, once your appetite decreases, the urge to binge on unhealthy foods automatically goes away. This in turn, reduces your food intake and makes it easier to stay in a calorie deficit.

Elimination of Harmful Foods

When you start following the juice cleanse, mos unhealthy foods like wheat, dairy, fermented foods, and gluten are automatically removed from your diet. It also significantly reduces your intake of alcohol and coffee When all such foods are eliminated from your usual diet you'll be left with healthy and wholesome foods. Also, the list of foods mentioned above are the primary sources o inflammation. By reducing the intake of inflammatory foods and replacing them with foods rich in antioxidants like fresh fruits and vegetables, you can improve you overall health. It also helps tackle inflammation, which i the primary cause of several painful and chronic health conditions. Once you take a break from consuming such harmful foods and then slowly start reintroducing then into your usual meals, it helps you understand the foods that suit and don't suit your body.

Conscious Food Choices

While following a juice cleanse, your intake of wholesome and fresh foods will increase. Since you will be consuming fresh juices after every couple of hours, your tummy will stay full. When your stomach is full, you will not spend all your time thinking about what your next meal will be. Once you feel satisfied, you can finally gain control over your eating habits. Making conscious food choices becomes easier when you start eating healthily.

Weight Loss

One of the most common reasons why a lot of people opt for a juice cleanse is because of the weight loss benefits it offers. If you feel like you are unable to lose weight regardless of how hard you exercise or are tired of trying diets that promise results but fail to deliver, then a juice cleanse will work. It not only enables you to feel more energetic but also triggers weight loss. A juice cleanse that lasts for a week is a great way to kick start any diet you want. It helps control your appetite and cravings in general but also reduces your calorie consumption. Even if your calorie intake reduces, your body gets all the nutrients it requires to stay healthy and energetic. When your calorie intake reduces, it becomes easier to maintain a calorie deficit. A calorie deficit is a precondition for weight loss. So, if you want to kickstart the process of weight loss, start a juice cleanse right away.

Plenty of Nutrition

A juice cleanse enables you to consume plenty of healthy fruits and vegetables. The diet of an average individual usually doesn't include plenty of fresh produce. When it comes to a juice cleanse, you will essentially be consuming only fruits and vegetables. This diet provides the body with not only all the vitamins and minerals it requires but also particular fiber and nutrients that kickstart internal cleaning and healing processes. Juices by nature include raw foods, and therefore, their nutrient composition stays the same. When you cook certain foods, their nutritional profile is disturbed. Well, this doesn't happen when you merely juice all the ingredients. Usually, vitamin B and other digestive and anti-inflammatory enzymes are destroyed during cooking processes. Since a juice cleanse bypasses all this, your body gets its share of nutrients and minerals.

Better Energy

Your body might take a day or two to get used to the new diet. During this period, it is a good idea to avoid drinking coffee or tea as you used to. You might even miss the constant snacking your earlier diet offered. However, once your body gets used to the new dietary regimen, you will start to feel more energetic than you ever did before. A juice cleanse refreshes your body and mind while giving it the break it needs.

Rehydration

The body of an average adult requires about eight glasses of water daily. Most of our bodies are usually dehydrated, and when this is combined with the consumption of diuretic beverages like tea or coffee, it only worsens the dehydration. By drinking sufficient fluids, your body can function more efficiently. Not only does your energy increase, but your body is also thoroughly rehydrated following a juice cleanse. Usually, people tend to feel a little sluggish and foggy late in the afternoon. To get over all this, try a juice cleanse. It provides your body with plenty of energy and nutrients while flushing out all the toxins present within.

Better Physical Health

A juice cleanse will certainly help enable you to feel better. Not just energy levels, but several chronic symptoms like blocked sinuses, headaches, general aches, rashes, bloating, and cramps tend to reduce. Most of the time, your body is usually trying to fight the things that we keep doing to it. It is especially true when it comes to food, and the lack of sleep, or inactivity. When you take a break and flood the system with nutrients and minerals, your energy levels will improve. Since a juice cleanse clears your system from within and enables all the essential organs to function optimally, you will feel better.

Cellular Healing

Once you switch to an organic plant-based diet, all the cells in your body start working optimally for re-establishing all the internal messaging and manufacturing processes. A combination of all these factors means that the mitochondria in all your cells start efficiently and effectively providing energy. They can do this without directing their precious energy towards fighting off a variety of free radicals and inflammation. It also reduces any blockages in the cells that prevent the DNA from functioning effectively.

Detoxification

Your body needs a variety of antioxidants and anti-inflammatory foods to support itself through all the phases of natural detoxification. As mentioned in the previous step, your body does have an internal system for detoxification. However, the system doesn't function optimally whenever there is an overload of toxins. By giving your body a break, all these systems get a chance to reset themselves. When you start consuming nutrient-dense foods, the way you would on the juice cleanse, your body gets all the support it requires to go through the different phases of detoxification. It also helps in the removal of the accumulated toxins stored within. It is one of the reasons why detox diets are suitable for your body.

Clear Skin

When your digestive system is overworked, it affects your skin health. When the toxic waste that kidneys have to deal with increases, they escape and start pouring out of the skin and result in blemishes and other skin troubles. By following a juice cleanse, your digestive health improves, but it also offers additional benefits. Consuming fruits and vegetables helps to cleanse the system from within while providing all the essential vitamins and minerals required to clear your skin. The simplest way to ensure you get sufficient fruits and vegetables is by following a juice cleanse. As mentioned, a juice cleanse helps in overall rehydration. Once your body is rehydrated, it helps improve your skin's health.

Now that you have gone through all the different benefits associated with a juice cleanse, you will realize it essentially resets your entire system. From improving your energy levels to clearing your digestive system and reducing inflammation, it gives your body a chance to concentrate on resting and repairing itself. By eliminating all sorts of unnecessary and unhealthy foods from your diet and replacing them with nutrient-dense foods, your body can get all the essential nutrients it needs for functioning optimally.

Note: Ensure that you are opting for organic ingredients whenever possible. Also, don't depend on prepackaged juices for this diet. Try to make the juices at home as often as you can, and it will improve the overall efficiency of this diet.

Chapter Four:

It's Natural to Worry - Answering All Your Juice Cleanse Questions

Common FAQs

A juice cleanse is probably quite different from your regular diet. Therefore, it is natural that you have particular questions and concerns. In this section, let us look at some of the most common questions people have before starting with a juice cleanse.

Can I do a juice cleanse if I am pregnant or breastfeeding?

When you are pregnant or breastfeeding, your body's energy and nutritional requirements increase. It is no ideal to try any diet during these stages. If your body doesn't get all the nutrients it requires, it cannot function optimally. It can also have an adverse effect on the growth of the fetus and milk production. Since the fetus depends on the mother's body for its nourishment, keep yourself well fed. Another reason why you must not attempt a juice cleanse while pregnant or breastfeeding is because this diet helps cleanse the system from within. It essentially means all the stored toxins are released into the bloodstream to eliminate them. This, in turn, increases the stress your body is already under during pregnancy.

Keep in mind that your body needs energy, not just to sustain itself and all the changes that occur, but it also requires the energy to support life growing within. So, any diet that reduces your calorie intake is never recommended. When you are breastfeeding, you might feel tired or sluggish. After pregnancy, it is quite likely that you might have put on a couple of pounds and would be keen on losing them as quickly as possible. However, it is not recommended to follow a juice cleanse, since it is not the ideal time for your body to release all the toxins stored within and place extra stress on itself. You also require additional calories to sustain your body while feeding the baby.

Is a juice cleanse safe for a diabetic?

If you have diabetes, then it is vital that you start a juice cleanse only under the strict supervision and guidance of your healthcare provider. Always opt for juices with a low glycemic index. Also, the nutritional and caloric requirements of an individual with diabetes will be quite different from those of a regular individual. Usually, a juice cleanse is not suggested for diabetics, but if your doctor allows you to, you can try it. However, if you notice any drastic fluctuations in your blood sugar levels, stop the diet, and seek medical help immediately.

I have a medical condition. Is a juice cleanse safe for me?

If you have any medical conditions like SIBO (small intestinal bacterial overgrowth) or gut dysbiosis, then juicing is not advisable. All the fermentable fiber present in juices tends to aggravate any gut disorders. Once again, don't forget to consult your doctor if you have any other medical conditions. Also, if you are just recovering from an eating disorder, major surgery, or are preparing for major surgery, avoid any diets, unless prescribed by your healthcare provider.

When should I try a juice cleanse?

You will need a couple of days to prepare yourself before you start a juice cleanse. Also, you will need a couple of days after the cleanse to get back to a healthy diet. It is easier to start this diet when you have a support system in place. Perhaps you could start it with your partner, friend, or maybe even a family member. Also, plan the diet so that you can relax during the initial three days of it. Since your body will be getting used to the diet during this period, it is always best to attempt it when you aren't under any stress.

Also, opt for such a time when you don't have any social commitments. It can become a little challenging to stick to this diet when you are planning a vacation, are on holiday, or have any other social obligations to attend. It becomes tricky to stick to the diet during holidays, and breaking your diet by drinking alcohol and consuming junk food is a recipe for disaster.

How much weight will I lose on a juice cleanse?

Weight loss is perhaps one of the most beneficial aspects of a juice cleanse. By resetting the eating habits and eliminating unnecessary cravings, it brings awareness to all the foods you consume. If you are trying to get a jumpstart on a healthier eating plan, then a juice will come in handy. Usually, you can lose anywhere between two to eight pounds on a one-week juice cleanse. However, weight loss differs from one person to another.

Can I exercise while on a juice cleanse?

Yes, you can exercise on a juice cleanse, but ensure that you don't engage in any high-intensity training. You can stick to light cardio and basic yoga. Keep in mind that a juice cleanse by itself is a physical event your body must endure. If you aren't careful and push yourself too hard, you will end up hurting yourself. Different forms of light exercise you can choose from include swimming, jogging, walking, hiking, or Pilates. All these exercises help stimulate your lymphatic moment while encouraging the detoxification of your body. If you do wish to exercise, ensure that you are consuming a sweet fruit juice immediately after the exercise session. If a specific juice tastes delicious, it means it has carbs, and these carbs are essential for replenishing the glycogen stores which are depleted during exercise.

Are there any risks involved in a juice cleanse?

There are a couple of risks involved with a juice cleanse, and they include instability in levels of blood sugar, foodborne illnesses from unpasteurized juices, lack of fiber, oxalate poisoning, difficulty managing weight, and improper fasting. If you have never tried a juice cleanse before, then fasting is a little tricky. Keep in mind that fasting is not for everyone. It is essential to be mindful of your sugar intake while on a juice cleanse. Your intake of fiber, fat, and protein will naturally reduce, while your intake of carbs and sugar can increase when you consume too many fruit juices. All the sugar will be readily absorbed into your bloodstream and can cause dramatic fluctuations in your blood sugar levels. Therefore, always consult your doctor before starting this diet. Consuming unpasteurized juices can compromise your immune system if you are not careful. Therefore, always wash the fruits and vegetables and peel their skins before making any juices.

Are there any side effects of a juice cleanse?

Juice cleanses offer plenty of benefits, but there are a couple of side effects you must be prepared for. Your body will take two or three days to get accustomed to the new diet. You might feel a little under the weather, experience mild headaches, minor skin blemishes, and some fatigue. These are all the common symptoms associated with detoxification, so don't be worried if you notice them. Keep in mind that these symptoms will soon go away once you get used to the new diet. Ensure that you drink plenty of water and keep your electrolyte levels balanced to avoid these side effects. Once your body is used to this diet, you can start reaping all the benefits associated with it, including healthy skin, better mood, improved digestion, and an overall sense of wellbeing.

Can I consume alcohol?

If you are interested in reaping all the benefits of a juice cleanse, then it's better you stay away from alcohol in all forms. Avoid alcohol during the preparation period, and the cleanse, too. Alcohol is a natural toxin that needs to pass through your liver. Since the idea of this diet is to give you a break, it is better to avoid ingesting any toxins.

Can I drink coffee?

Coffee is highly acidic and contains plenty of caffeine in it. To make the most of this cleanse, avoid consuming coffee. If you are used to frequently drinking coffee, then it would be better to slowly wean yourself off or drastically reduce your intake in the weeks or days building up to the cleanse. Doing this helps because you can easily circumvent any potential symptoms associated with a lack of caffeine. If you think you will not be able to entirely eliminate caffeine from your diet, it might be a good idea to move from traditional coffee to something more organic like herbal teas, or a less acidic brew of coffee.

Can I expect any changes to my urine/stools?

It is highly unlikely that your bowel movements will be irregular, and you don't have to worry about spending more time on the toilet than usual. However, the urge to urinate will be more frequent since you will be consuming a liquid diet. You might also experience a little constipation during the initial phase. You don't have to panic if that's the case. Since the average bulk of your meals is going to reduce considerably, the output will also be less. After consulting your doctor, you can take colonic or Senna pills to help along the process of excretion.

Will I get sufficient fiber on a juice cleanse?

A juice cleanse is designed such that it gives your digestive system a break to expedite the internal cleansing and detoxification process. Keep in mind that juices don't usually contain large amounts of fiber. Whenever you consume large amounts of fiber, your body has to break this down and uses some energy to do so. When the need for this process is eliminated, all the energy it would have used for digesting fiber will be directed towards detoxification.

Will I get sufficient protein on a juice cleanse?

You don't have to worry about your protein intake while on a juice cleanse. If you are mindful of the types of juices you consume, your body will get all the protein it requires. However, one problem you might run into is that most of the food sources that are rich in protein are usually not appetizing to drink like broccoli, asparagus, and cauliflower. There are certain types of juices like the ones made with watermelon, bananas, carrots, oranges, and strawberries that can provide sufficient protein. About 10 to 35% of your daily calorie intake must be from proteins. So, you need about 50 to 175 grams of protein in your daily diet. One serving of dates has 3 grams of protein, oranges have 1 gram of protein, strawberries have 1 gram, and watermelon has 2 grams of protein.

Can I eat during a juice cleanse?

If you are interested in reaping all the benefits offered by a juice cleanse, then avoid consuming any solid foods during this period. Avoid snacking altogether. When your body starts using its energy for digesting the food you consume, the effects of a juice cleansing tend to slow down. If you have to eat something, then always opt for organic vegetables, fruits, soaked nuts, or some seeds. Some simple foods you can include are cucumber, celery, bananas, avocados, sprouted or soaked almonds, carrots, and apples. For best results, it is advised that you stick to only one food at any given time. Keep in mind that the idea of a juice cleanse is to give your digestive system a break. If you keep eating during the cleanse, it will prove to be counterproductive.

What can I do if I feel low in energy?

Whenever you make a dietary change, you will notice fluctuations in your energy levels until your body gets used to the new diet. The same holds true for a juice cleanse, too. Therefore, don't be worried if you notice any reduction in your energy levels during the first two days. It is not only normal, but you must expect it as well. Even if a dietary change doesn't seem like a big deal to you, it certainly is a big deal for your body. So, be patient and give yourself a while to get used to the diet. Once your body gets acclimated to this diet, your energy levels will stabilize, and you will feel more energetic than ever before.

All this happens because your internal organs are working very hard to clean and rejuvenate themselves during this break that you have given them in the form of a juice cleanse. If you can power through this period, and relax a little, you can enjoy all the different benefits it offers. Whenever you start feeling a little low on energy, take a break and lie down on your back for a couple of minutes.

Can I take supplements on a juice cleanse?

If you are used to taking a regular multivitamin, you can stick to it. However, you don't necessarily have to take a multivitamin since most of the juices you consume will have all the nutrients and vitamins your body requires. If you take any other supplements for vitamin B1 or omega-3 fatty acids, keep taking those since a juice cleanse doesn't provide these specific nutrients. Always consult your doctor before you make any changes to the supplements you consume.

Will I gain weight after the cleanse?

You will lose all the water weight your body has been holding onto during a juice cleanse. If weight loss is your priority, then you must have a maintenance plan to keep up the weight loss. You might not gain all the weight immediately after a cleanse. However, some of the water weight you lost during the diet might return. A juice cleanse helps reset all your dietary habits and makes you conscious of the foods you consume. If you follow a healthy dietary schedule once the cleanse ends, you can maintain the weight loss. You will learn more about this in the subsequent chapters.

Should I use a variety of juices?

Ensure that you include a variety of juices to your daily diet, or else you will soon get bored of it. Since juice will be the only form of nutrition you'll be consuming, there must be variety. It can get rather tiring and boring if you have to drink the same juice throughout the day for seven days in a row. Use the different recipes given in this book, or follow the sample juice cleanse plan to get started.

How long does fresh juice last?

If there is any pulp leftover in the juice, then you must consume it immediately. Exposure to heat or oxygen during juicing can alter the nutritional profile of the juice. If the juice is cold-pressed, then it eliminates nutrient damage caused due to heat or oxygen exposure during the juicing process. However, even cold-pressed juices can degrade in their nutritional value due to the presence of bacteria, yeast, or mold. Therefore, try to consume the juice as soon as it is made or within 24-hours, provided it is properly refrigerated. The flavor of the juice might change when it is refrigerated.

Can I freeze fresh fruit juices?

If you cannot immediately consume the juices after making them, you can freeze them for consumption later on. However, avoid doing this as much as possible. If you have to freeze them, then slightly unscrew the lid and take a sip to make space for expansion once the juice freezes. You then simply need to defrost the juice in a bowl of warm water, and it is ready for consumption. Keep in mind the appearance and the texture of the juice.

How do I store fresh juice?

As mentioned earlier, you should drink the juice immediately for optimal nutritional benefits. However, if you have to store it, always place it in an airtight container and keep it in the refrigerator. Try to consume it as soon as you possibly can and no later than 24-hours.

Should I wash the fruits and vegetables before juicing?

Ensure that you thoroughly wash the fruits and vegetables before juicing. You can wash them in a solution made of lemon juice and saltwater to remove traces of any pesticides or preservatives. Once you clean them with this solution, don't forget to rinse them before adding them to the juice thoroughly. Also, some certain fruits and vegetables have to be peeled before juicing. If you don't peel them, then all the pesticides and chemicals present in their peel will be absorbed by your body.

Note: A juice cleanse is safe for an average healthy adult, but if you are breastfeeding, pregnant, or have any other health complications, don't attempt it right away. If you have any pre-existing health conditions, always check with your healthcare provider.

Now that you've gone through the list of FAQs and answers, you should feel better about a juice cleanse.

Chapter Five:

To Juice or To Blend?

Which One Is Right for Your

Cleanse?

Juicing vs. Blending

One question that might pop into your head as you consider a juice cleanse is whether you should be juicing or blending. The terms juicing and blending might be used synonymously, but they are quite different from one another. The primary difference between these two is that blended drinks like smoothies contain plenty of fiber whereas juices contain hardly any fiber.

Let's look more closely at the differences between them.

Juicing

Juicing is a process that helps extract all the water and nutrients present in ingredients. During this process, indigestible fiber is automatically eliminated in the form of pulp. Without all this fiber, it becomes easier for your digestive system to break down and digest the foods you consume. It also assists in better absorption of all the nutrients. Since the idea of a juice cleanse is about giving your digestive system a break, juicing will come in handy. Juicing ensures that plenty of nutrients are readily available to your body in larger quantities than if you were to consume all the raw ingredients individually. After all, it takes about two minutes to drink a glass of juice. On the other hand, it can take you 10 minutes to eat an entire apple.

It will come in handy if you have a sensitive digestive system or any health condition that prevents your body from effectively and efficiently processing the fiber you consume. The fiber present in vegetable and fruit juices can slow down the digestive process long enough to provide a steady stream of nutrients that are released into your bloodstream. It is one of the reasons why you tend to feel full while on a juice cleanse, even when you don't consume any solid food.

Whenever fiber is removed from fruits and vegetables, the liquid juices are readily absorbed into your bloodstream. If you are drinking only fruit juices, keep in mind that it can cause significant fluctuations in your blood sugar levels. Any instability in your blood sugar levels can affect your overall mood and energy levels.

Juicing helps create a smooth drink since all the fiber from the produce is already extracted.

Blending

On the other hand, smoothies tend to contain the entire fruit or vegetable, including the peel, pulp, and everything else. So, all the fiber present in the fruits and vegetables stays intact. However, during the blending process, the fiber present in fruits and vegetables is broken, and it makes it easier to digest. Apart from this, it also helps create a slow and steady release of nutrients into the bloodstream to avoid any fluctuations in the levels of blood sugar. Smoothies are usually more filling since they contain all the fiber. They are certainly quicker to make when compared to juices. So, a smoothie is a great way to start your day. A smoothie can be a filling breakfast or a delicious snack.

The volume of the end product you make will certainly increase when all the fiber is present in the smoothie. Also, you can add more portions of vegetables and fruits into a single serving of smoothie than into a juice. To make a smoothie, you merely need to toss in your favorite fruits, vegetables, and add some liquid to it and then blend. Once it is thoroughly blended, you'll be left with a rich and creamy drink.

However, there is one aspect of smoothie that a lot of people tend to forget. Even if you don't have to chew the smoothie, your stomach still has to digest it thoroughly. There is plenty of fiber left in a smoothie that your stomach has to absorb. On a juice cleanse, the idea is to give your stomach a break, so a smoothie might not be the best choice.

Fiber

Fiber is vital for efficient digestion and absorption of nutrients. Therefore, it is essential for your overall well being. Juices don't really contain plenty of fiber. Fiber comes in two forms: soluble fiber and insoluble fiber. Soluble fiber is the fiber present in carrots, peas, citrus fruits, apples, and green beans. This fiber, as the name suggests, gets easily dissolved in water and helps slow down the process of digestion. This, in turn, helps regulate your blood sugar levels. On the other hand, insoluble fiber is the one that's present in vegetables like dark leafy vegetables, cruciferous vegetables, and potatoes. Insoluble fiber essentially bulks up your bowel movement while stimulating more action in the intestinal tract.

Nutrients

Whenever you convert vegetables and fruits into juices, all the nutrients present in them are more concentrated. Not just this, but your body can readily absorb them. It is primarily because a significant chunk of these vitamins and minerals that are found within fruits are typically in the juice and not the fibrous material or the pulp present in a smoothie.

Antioxidants

Fiber and other phytochemicals like antioxidant

compounds are present in vegetable and fruit pulp. Juices also contain phytochemicals to a certain extent, but blended smoothies tend to have more of these phytochemicals. So, in this regard, blended fruits and vegetables tend to have a higher concentration of helpful compounds like antioxidants. Since these are primarily present in the fibrous membrane of the fruit like the pulp and the peel, consuming smoothies will be beneficial. That being said, it is not fair to downplay the different antioxidants present in fruit juices.

Digestion

All those who support juicing suggest that consumption of fruits and vegetables without any fiber makes it easier for your body to digest it. Also, consuming juices enhances your body's ability to absorb all the nutrients present in it. Beta-carotene is a helpful carotenoid that is derived from juiced produce instead of whole food forms. In an analysis, it was confirmed that juicing helps increase the levels of beta-carotene in the blood. It is believed that high levels of beta-carotene in the blood is directly linked with a lower risk of cancer.

It has been suggested that soluble fibers decrease the absorption of beta-carotene in blood by about 30 to 50%. Still, even if there is fiber present in smoothies, the cell walls of the ingredients are fundamentally broken down, which, in turn, improves your body's ability to absorb beta-carotene. However, be mindful of your intake of fiber. If your diet is completely devoid of fiber, then it will do your body more harm than good.

Sugar

One thing you must always watch out for regardless of whether you want to drink juice or a smoothie is the sugar present in it. Smoothies and juices can both elevate your sugar levels, but the effect is more dramatic and rapid when you drink juices. Since juices are more concentrated than smoothies, all the sugar present in them is quickly absorbed into the bloodstream. On the other hand, when you blend fruits or vegetables, you start to feel full quite quickly. All the pulp, fiber, and peel present increase the volume of the drink, which, in turn, helps you instantly feel full while reducing your total calorie intake. For instance, you will end up with one glass of juice after juicing two oranges.

Weight Loss

When it comes to weight loss, juices are the better option. However, it would not be fair to consider juice to be the holy grail of weight loss. It essentially depends on your daily lifestyle, dietary regimen, and maintenance plan. If you eat healthily, add some exercise and live an active lifestyle, then juicing is a great way to maintain your weight loss. Juicing is also a great way to kickstart weight loss. For instance, if you have overindulged on calories over the weekend or have been eating unhealthy for a while now, then a juice cleanse is a great idea to get back on track. Prolonged periods of inactivity, coupled with constant snacking, can lead to weight gain. To rectify this, use a juice cleanse.

Decision Time

Juicing offers a variety of benefits, and perhaps the mos significant benefit it offers is the higher concentration o all the nutrients. It indirectly increases your consumptior of vegetables and fruits while enhancing your body's ability to absorb nutrients. It comes in handy, especially i you have a tough time eating fruits and vegetables or their own. On the downside, you might miss out on the essential fibers present in whole fruits and vegetables Apart from that, you also miss out on crucial compound present in the pulp. When it comes to blending, you pretty much get everything a vegetable or fruit offers However, some people are put off by the texture of pulp.

Now that you are aware of the meaning of blending anc juicing, and the different aspects involved in each, the decision is entirely up to you.

There is one stipulation you cannot ignore when it come to both blending and juicing, and that is the sugar presen in them. If weight loss is your priority, then you must pa attention to the sugar you consume either directly o indirectly. You can, however, minimize spikes in blooc sugar levels by adding different sources of fat, fiber, anc protein to the juices like avocados, protein powder unsweetened Greek yogurt, or even Chia seeds.

Rules

Only certain fruits and vegetables should be combinec

together. Fruits and vegetables on their own offer plenty of nutritional value, but a combination of some can affect your digestive enzymes. You don't have to worry about this in green juices and smoothies, but certain vegetables with high starch content like broccoli, carrots, zucchini, and beetroot don't combine well with all sorts of foods. Starchy foods should be consumed separately since the enzymes required to digest starches are different from the ones used for any other food group. Therefore, you should stick with the various recipes given in this book since they have been designed keeping the requirements of a juice cleanse in mind.

Another simple rule you must keep in mind is to not leave the juice exposed to air. In fact, make it a point to consume it within 15 minutes. If you think you cannot drink it right away, store it in an airtight container and place it in the refrigerator until you are ready. However, as mentioned in the previous chapter, don't allow any juice or smoothie to stay in the refrigerator for more than 24 hours.

Right Equipment

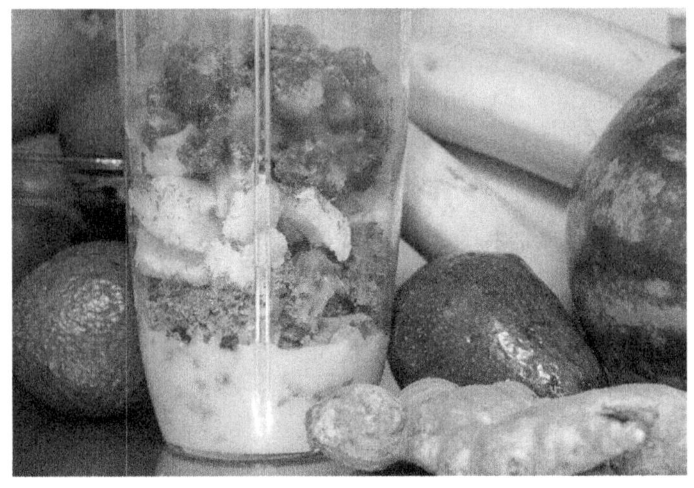

To get the maximum nutrition from the juices and smoothies you make, you must use the right equipment. It is a good idea to invest in a high-quality juicer. Most of the cheaper centrifugal juicers expose all the ingredients to heat and oxygen during the juicing process. This kind of exposure tends to destroy helpful nutrients and enzymes present in the ingredients. The upfront cost of a good quality juicer or a premium cold press juicer might be high, but it is an investment that keeps on giving. The extraction process in a centrifugal juicer is quite rough when compared to cold press juicers that tend to thoroughly press and squeeze vegetables and fruits while providing clear juice. The same stands true for a blender as well. The blender must be gentle so that it doesn't heat any of the enzymes present in the ingredients or start pulling apart the digestive fiber. We all certainly splurge on different things like clothes, shoes, bags and so on. Now might be a good time to splurge on proper kitchen equipment if it helps improve your overall health.

By now, you would have realized that blending and juicing are entirely different processes altogether. There certainly are some arguments in favor of both of these techniques. However, when it comes to a juice cleanse, juicing is a favorable option. Since your body no longer has to spend any energy to digest fiber, it can take a break from its usual functions and use this time for resting itself. Also, when you choose fruits or vegetables, all the nutrients present in it can be easily absorbed by your body. Since it doesn't have to spend any energy on absorption, all its focus can be shifted towards detoxifying and cleansing itself.

Chapter Six:

Preparation Is the Key to Success- Getting Ready to Start Your Juice Cleanse

Understand Yourself

To successfully start and complete a juice cleanse, it is essential that you prepare yourself. Unless you dedicate a couple of days to prepare your body and mind for the juice cleanse, you cannot maximize the benefits it offers. Also, your overall experience will be more pleasant, and you can avoid any of the potential side effects associated with a juice cleanse by preparing yourself in the days leading up to the cleanse. Usually, it is recommended that you allocate anywhere between 2 to 7 days for a pre-cleanse routine. The time taken mainly depends on your usual lifestyle and eating habits. Here are a few categories for you to consider. Decide which describes you the best and follow the appropriate recommendations for the pre-cleanse diet.

Category One

This category primarily consists of all those who can be termed as health enthusiasts. If you are used to eating a healthy diet but have gone off track, then the usual reset period is anywhere between 1 to 2 days. If your typical meals consist of healthy and wholesome foods without any junk or foods devoid of nutrients, then you fall under this category.

Category Two

If you usually eat well during the week but like to allocate a cheat day for the weekends, then your aim must be to make healthy eating habits more consistent. Before you start a juice cleanse, spend at least 3 to 4 days in the precleanse state. It helps eliminate any remnants of processed foods, caffeine, and alcohol from your body.

Category Three

If your usual diet consists of prepackaged and processed foods, and you don't consume sufficient fresh foods or plant-based foods, then your pre-cleanse stage will last longer. If you want to avoid any unpleasant symptoms of detox, then it is important that you spend at least five days in the pre-cleanse diet stage.

Category Four

If you love fast food and cannot imagine a meal without sugary treats or other junk food, then you belong in this category. Before you attempt a juice cleanse, it is important that you allow your energy levels, attitude, metabolic, and digestive system to stabilize. To do this, you will need to stick to the pre-cleanse diet for a week. You can spend more time in this stage since it effectively improves your ability to follow through a juice cleanse. Apart from this, it also reduces the chances of experiencing any of the unpleasant symptoms associated with a detox diet.

Pre-Cleanse Regime

Now that you're aware of how long an ideal pre-cleanse must last let us look at what a pre-cleanse regime looks like.

Reduce Stimulants

If you want to make the most of the benefits offered by a juice cleanse, then it is quite essential to reduce the consumption of any stimulants. Usual stimulants include caffeine, alcohol, or nicotine. If you are used to drinking or smoking regularly, then it is time to start eliminating these two things from your usual routine. Not only are they harmful to your health, but they wreak havoc on your body's metabolism too. Now, let us come to the third culprit: caffeine. If you are used to drinking coffee or soda regularly, it is time you take steps to wean yourself off these highly caffeinated and acidic beverages before you start a juice cleanse. If you think you won't be able to get through your day without a cup of coffee, then instead of a highly acidic variety, opt for lower acid or cold brew coffee. You can even try decaf instead of regular coffee.

Increase Hydration

The simplest way to cleanse your body is by drinking water. Usually, people tend to mistake dehydration for hunger. When your cells are thoroughly hydrated, it eliminates the chance of false hunger pangs. One of the most important steps towards preparing yourself for a juice cleanse is hydrating your body. It also helps start the process of flushing away toxins.

Increase Intake of Vegetables and Fruits

The simplest way to increase your intake of digestive enzymes is by consuming more fruits and vegetables. In fact, start adding a couple of fruit and vegetable juices to your daily diet. It is a great way to introduce the idea of a juice cleanse to your body. By gradually increasing your intake of liquids and cutting away solid food, it prepares your body for the seven-day juice cleanse.

Avoid Processed Foods

Processed foods are not suitable for your health. Regardless of what the labels claim, they are harmful. They contain plenty of additives, colorants, and are devoid of all essential nutrients. The sooner you stop eating such foods, the sooner you can improve your overall health. Before you purchase anything, ensure that you carefully read through the label. If there is an ingredient on the label that you don't recognize or cannot pronounce, chances are, your body doesn't know it either. Instead of increasing the toxic burden, try reducing it. Whenever you purchase any produce, ensure that it is organic. By following this simple routine, you can ensure that your body starts its detoxification process. Most processed foods are rich in unhealthy carbs, sugars, and fats. These foods are unhealthy, but they are quite addictive. So, give yourself some time to get over these addictions. Once you do this, it becomes easier to follow a juice cleanse.

Avoid Animal Products

A day or two before the pre-cleanse routine starts, make a commitment to yourself to consume a plant-based diet. This essentially means you must avoid all animal products like meat, eggs, dairy, or even honey. If you are usually used to consuming animal products daily, then make it a point to not eat any more than once a week. Consumption of animal products increases the stress on your digestive system. The best way to reduce the burden on your digestive system is by providing it with food, it can easily break down. Therefore, increase the consumption of plant-based foods while avoiding animal-based foods altogether.

Sleep

Regardless of how hectic your life gets, ensure that you get at least 6 to 8 hours of good quality and undisturbed sleep every night. It is not just the duration of the sleep, but the quality of the sleep that matters. Unless your body gets sufficient rest, it cannot get used to the new diet. Lack of sleep, coupled with a significant dietary change, acts as a stressor for your body. When your body is stressed, its fight or flight response is triggered. In this stage, it doesn't promote weight loss and, instead, concentrates on preserving you. When stress increases, it promotes the release of cortisol, which only worsens the symptoms of stress you experience. Since the idea of a pre-cleanse is easing your body into a new diet, ensure that you give your body the rest it needs.

Exercise

You merely need to tweak your exercise routine to match your energy levels during the pre-cleanse stage. Since you will be making dietary changes, don't over train and don't exert yourself unnecessarily. If you do this, you will essentially burn yourself out before the diet even starts. So, start listening to your body and stop exercising whenever it feels like it is getting to be too much. If you keep using during the pre-cleanse stage, it prepares your body for exercising during the juice cleanse, also.

Attitude

Don't forget to set an intention for the juice cleanse you wish to follow. An intention is a commitment you are making to yourself to changing a specific part of your life that no longer serves your overall well being. What are the goals that you wish to attain using a juice cleanse? Is there a specific aspect of your life you wish to heal? How will you know if you have successfully accomplished your goals? Spend some time and think about these questions. Your answers will reveal your motivation for starting the diet. This reason will ensure that you stay on track and complete the 7-day juice cleanse without giving up.

Supplements

If a healthcare professional has prescribed a specific supplement because of any diagnosed deficiency you have, then keep taking it. You don't need any special supplements for a juice cleanse. If you are used to taking a multivitamin, then you can stick to it. Consuming probiotics, supplements, omega-3 fatty acids, and multivitamins will undoubtedly come in handy while doing a juice cleanse. Usually, your intake of macronutrients and certain micronutrients like protein, fiber, fats, vitamin D, vitamin E, zinc, vitamin B12, selenium, and omega-3 fatty acids decreases while on a juice cleanse. Well, your usual diet also plays a significant role here. Depending upon what your typical diet looks like, your nutrient needs will vary.

Probiotics

Your gut microbiome or the bacteria present in your gut plays an essential role in your overall well being. It not only affects your digestive health, but your overall mood, energy, the health of your skin, and your body's immune response. Whenever you think of bacteria, you might imagine something harmful. However, the gut microbiome is quintessential for your health. Therefore, maintaining the health of this beneficial microflora is essential. The gut microbiome helps your body digest and absorb nutrients present in the food. It also helps produce crucial vitamins like vitamins B and K while suppressing the growth of other harmful microorganisms. The best way to maintain the health of this helpful bacteria is by feeding them probiotics.

The best sources of probiotic foods you can add to your diet are yogurt, sauerkraut, miso, kombucha, kefir, kimchi, tempeh, buttermilk, pickles, and natto. The most common types of probiotics include Lactobacillus, Bifidobacterium, and Saccharomyces boulardii. Always consult your healthcare provider before you add any probiotic supplements to your daily diet. You don't have to do this if you are experimenting with probiotic foods, but supplements work differently and are more targeted.

Multivitamin

Stress, poor sleep patterns, or any dietary deficiencies can present themselves in the form of nutritional deficiencies. To avoid all this, you can take a multivitamin supplement. Multivitamin supplements can improve your overall health. They usually contain calcium, vitamin D, vitamin B, magnesium, vitamin C, zinc, and antioxidants. Calcium and vitamin D help improve your bone health. Folic acid reduces birth defects, magnesium helps relax your body, vitamin B12 improves your overall energy levels and cognitive functioning, and vitamin C and zinc strengthen your immune response. These are just some of the benefits offered by multivitamins.

Multivitamins are certainly essential supplements since they ensure your body gets all the vital vitamins. However, keep in mind that every human body is unique and its health care needs are quite different. Never use a one size fits all kind of approach while tackling any health issues. It is one of the reasons why the multivitamin supplement you take must be ideal for your body. There are certain supplements you can take to improve specific areas of your health. For instance, taking a supplement of omega-3 fatty acids help regulate levels of high triglycerides. Therefore, always consult your healthcare provider to find the right dosage and the kind of multivitamin supplement you must be taking. Also, if you have any pre-existing health condition or are on any medication, consult your doctor. Specific multivitamins have an adverse effect when they mingle with particular medications. Whenever you look for a multivitamin, make sure that it's natural, highly bioavailable, and made without any artificial colors. Also, it has no fillers, additives, and is free of allergens.

Omega-3 Fatty Acids

Omega-3 fatty acids can help improve your overall health and cognitive functioning. It is believed that these fatty acids help tackle anxiety or depression, improve the liver's health, promote the brain's health, reduce the risk of heart diseases, reduce any symptoms of metabolic syndrome, fight inflammation, tackle autoimmune responses, improve bone or joint health, and alleviate menstrual pain. Consuming an omega-3 fatty acid supplement is a good idea. Since most diets are usually devoid of this essential nutrient, a supplement will come in handy. The best source of omega-3 fatty acids is from the consumption of naturally fatty fish. The best sources of omega-3 fatty acids supplements include natural fish oil, mammalian oil, krill oil, algal oil, processed fish oil, omega-3 capsules, green-lipped mussel oil, and ALA oil.

If you want the juice cleanse to be successful, then preparation is essential. Always plan the juices you wish to make, and ensure that you have all the ingredients ready. If you want to make all the juices at home, then you will require a juicer. It is always better to make the juices at home since it gives you absolute control over the ingredients you consume and the quantity. To support the nutrition you get from the juice cleanse, you might have to add a few supplements. However, don't add any supplements before consulting your doctor or healthcare provider. Apart from this, start eliminating certain harmful foods from your diet to make it easier for your body to get accustomed to a juice cleanse.

Chapter Seven:

Now You're Ready to Cleanse... What Does A Typical Day Look Like?

During the Cleanse

Now that you have successfully completed the pre-cleanse, it is time for the juice cleanse. In this section, let us look at certain simple things you must keep in mind while following a juice cleanse. By sticking to this advice, you can optimize the benefits offered by a juice cleanse.

Diet

If you want to fully reap the benefits of a juice cleanse, it is essential that you avoid consuming solid food. If you eat anything during this cleanse, it merely slows down the benefits it offers. Apart from this, it also exerts certain stress on the digestive system. Since a juice cleanse is performed with the basic idea of giving a break to your internal mechanisms, the consumption of solid food is not advisable. However, if you feel the need to eat, you can opt for organic fruits, vegetables, or even soaked seeds and nuts.

Exercise

While on a juice cleanse, try restricting the level of physical activity to something quite light or mild. Simple exercises you can perform without straining yourself are walking, yoga, or basic stretching. While on a juice cleanse, be prepared for certain changes in your energy levels. It merely means your body is getting used to the diet. So, start paying close attention to what your body requires and don't push yourself beyond the breaking limit. There is a popular misconception that high-intensity training, coupled with extremely low levels of calorie intake, speed up the process of weight loss. Well, you might lose a couple of pounds initially, but then the weight loss will stop. If your calorie expenditure is way beyond what your body can sustain, your body shifts into starvation mode. In this mode, you will not lose any weight, and instead, your body starts accumulating fat.

Activities

Whenever you are on a juice cleanse, you can use this time for indulging in various other productive activities. Perhaps you can concentrate on your work, provided it doesn't stress you out too much. Apart from that, it is also the perfect time to spend some time indulging in your hobbies. If you don't have a hobby, then there is no time like the present to pick up a new one. If there's something you have been meaning to do, then now the right time for it. You can also use this time for some introspection. You can write in a journal, go for walks, meditate for a while, or even listen to soothing music. Try to avoid any places that are crowded and noisy. During the juice cleanse, you might notice your senses are more sensitive than usual. Ensure that you have plenty of free time to take care of yourself.

Lemon and Water

The citric acid present in lemon juice is an incredible natural stimulant. As soon as you wake up in the morning, avoid reaching for a regular cup of coffee. Instead, grab a glass of warm water, and squeeze some lemon juice into it. Drink this concoction before you drink anything else. The enzymes present in the lemon juice help stimulate your liver and kickstart the cleansing process even before you start drinking juices. This is one simple ritual that has numerous health benefits. It is also believed to improve your body's metabolism and assist in weight loss. Therefore, this is one ritual you must add to your daily routine, regardless of whether you are on a juice cleanse or not.

Consistency

Ensure that you are consuming juices after every 2 to 2 ½ hours. The gap between two consecutive juices must not be more than this. Consistency is key when it comes to a juice cleanse. Thinking about drinking 6 to 8 juices daily might sound like a lot. However, when you space it out over 12 hours, it is not that much. You will essentially be having your last juice of the day two hours before you fall asleep. If you don't stick to the schedule, then it is quite likely that you will start feeling hungry, and it can result in a drastic decline in your blood sugar levels. So, even if you're not hungry, stick to the schedule. If there are any drastic fluctuations in your blood sugar levels, it will affect the overall efficiency of the diet while adversely affecting your mood.

Tips for Detox

If you want to improve the overall efficiency of the juice cleanse, then here are some additional tips you can try.

Dry Brushing

Dry brushing is a very simple technique you can add to your usual wellness routine. It helps tighten your skin, reduce cellulite, engage your lymphatic system, improve digestion, and encourage detoxification of your body. There are so many benefits associated with a simple regimen.

Upward strokes, coupled with the friction of dry brushing, help invigorate your lymphatic system, which, in turn, enables detoxification while filling your body with more energy. Whenever you select a brush for dry brushing, ensure that it is the right fit for you. Brushes with a hand strap work well if you have decent flexibility. If you think you're not flexible, then opt for a brush that has a more extended handle for accessing any of the hard to reach places. Always look for brushes made of natural instead of synthetic fibers. The bristles of the brush must be stiff and firm; however, if you have sensitive skin, these kinds of bristles might end up scratching your skin. So, always start with a softer brush. Once your skin gets used to dry brushing, you can opt for a stiffer brush.

Ensure that the technique you use meets your overall mood. For instance, quick strokes can be invigorating, whereas slow and rhythmic strokes have calming energy. So, depending upon whether you want to make yourself feel more energetic or wish to calm yourself down, the strokes you use must be different. While dry brushing, ensure that all the strokes you make move towards your heart. You can always place a towel on the ground before you start dry brushing or maybe even stand in the bathtub. Keep applying light but constant pressure while dry brushing.

Always start by dry brushing your feet, then move upward towards the calves, then thighs, then the stomach, your back, chest, and arms. Make sure that you stroke each area at least three times, and all the strokes must be directed towards your heart. Perhaps the simplest way to end this ritual is by rinsing in the shower or moisturizing your body. It helps enhance the look of your detoxified skin while giving it the moisture it requires.

Sweating it Out

Whenever you sweat, your body tends to remove toxins. So, if you can sweat a lot, your body starts effectively flushing out all the toxins. Therefore, one way to speed up the process of detoxification is by sweating it out. Perhaps you can sit in a sauna or even engage in any quick aerobic exercise that makes you sweat. You can go for a brisk walk or maybe jump rope for 10 minutes. By doing this, your body starts generating heat on a cellular level. This way, it speeds up the process of detoxification. However, while doing this, be careful that you are not overexerting or overtiring yourself. Keep in mind that your body is on a cleanse, and your energy levels might not have stabilized yet.

Eliminating Waste

As you progress through the juice cleanse, don't be surprised if you see a reduction in elimination. When it comes to a juice cleanse, less in equals less out. However, don't ever overlook any of the signals your body tries to give you. If you start experiencing any detox symptoms like nausea but haven't yet eliminated any waste from the intestines, then you might need to stimulate elimination using an herbal laxative like Senna or a colonic enema. If this feeling of constipation doesn't go away, stop the diet, and seek medical help immediately.

Detox Bath

Regardless of whether you are trying to alleviate any symptoms of detox or are following a juice cleanse, following the simple detoxifying ritual will undoubtedly improve how you feel. Every day, our bodies are constantly exposed to a variety of toxins. Some of these toxins are within our control, but most of them are out of our control. You can certainly do your best, and opt for organic food, use natural homemade beauty products, filter the water you consume, and so on. However, most of the toxins we are exposed to are external and uncontrollable. As mentioned in the previous chapters, our bodies have an internal mechanism for eliminating all the toxins that are stored. However, your body is not a tireless machine, and even it needs a break. Therefore, incorporate a simple self-care regimen like a detox bath to enable your body to metabolize all the toxic waste quickly. Once your body is thoroughly detoxed, you can lead a healthier and happier life.

Here's a simple detoxifying recipe for a ginger detox bath. This recipe includes Epsom salts. Epsom salts are also known as magnesium sulfate. They essentially help remove all toxins, reduce stress, soothe soreness, regulate the activity of enzymes, improve the quality of sleep, enhance your body's ability to absorb nutrients, and benefit the circulatory system. The baking soda used in this recipe helps in neutralizing any of the hard chemicals present in tap water while enabling your body to absorb the nutrients within. By adding apple cider vinegar, it helps ease any body aches and enables your body to maintain the alkalinity it desires. The ginger present in it warms up your body and helps you sweat. When you start sweating, your body starts expelling toxins through sweat.

Let us look at the recipe for this simple ginger detox bath.

Combine half a cup of Epsom salts with half a cup of baking soda and half a cup of apple cider vinegar. To this, add two tablespoons of ground ginger. If you don't have ground ginger, you can substitute it with two ginger tea bags. Once you have combined all this, add it to a lukewarm bath and simply soak in it. Allow the properties of all these ingredients to get to work.

Note: This recipe is good for one soak. If you want to make the bath more intense, you merely need to double up on all the quantities. If you want, you can also replace ginger with any other essential oil that you like. Perhaps you can use lavender, jasmine, rose, or any other essential oil you want. Various essential oils have different properties. For instance, lavender is commonly used for its soothing and calming properties, whereas peppermint is quite invigorating. Merely substitute the ginger used in the above-mentioned recipe with any of the essential oil you want.

By following these simple tips for detoxification, you can assist your body in its internal detoxification. The juice cleanse helps detoxify your body from within, and these different techniques will effectively speed up this process.

Typical Day

As soon as you wake up in the morning, the first thing you must drink is a mix of lukewarm water with some freshly squeezed lemon juice. One glass of this mix will kickstart the functioning of your digestive system and prepare it for the rest of the day.

- 8 to 9 am: It is time for a refreshing juice made of green leafy vegetables.
- 10:30 to 11 am: You can opt for a juice or a smoothie.
- 1 to 2 pm: You can opt for a juice or a smoothie. If you crave something filling, then a smoothie will help.
- 3 to 4 pm: It is time for a re-energizing juice like one made with beetroots, carrots, and apples.
- 5 to 6 pm: You can opt for a juice or a smoothie.
- 6 to 8 pm: You can opt for a smoothie, or some almond/ cashew/ or any other nut-based milk.

Ensure that the last juice or smoothie you consume is about 2 hours before bedtime. This gives your body sufficient time to digest the juice you consume.

7-Day Sample Plan

Monday

Wake up

8 to 9 am: Green detox juice

10:30 to 11am: Antioxidant boost juice

1 to 2 pm: Green protein boost juice

3 to 4pm: Ginger-beet juice

5 to 6pm: Dandelion green juice

6 to 8pm: Heart-healthy juice

Tuesday

8 to 9 am: The green machine

10:30 to 11am: Powerful antioxidant juice

1 to 2 pm: Protein powerhouse green juice

3 to 4pm: Beetroot juice

5 to 6pm: Liver cleansing juice

6 to 8pm: The cholesterol fighter

Wednesday

8 to 9 am: Natural energy green juice

10:30 to 11am: Kidney detox juice

1 to 2 pm: Green sprouts juice

3 to 4pm: Mellow matter juice

5 to 6pm: Liver scrubber juice

6 to 8pm: Vegetable juice

Thursday

8 to 9 am: Electric green juice

10:30 to 11am: Kidney cleanse juice

1 to 2 pm: Tomato and alfalfa juice

3 to 4pm: Tropical carrot-apple juice

5 to 6pm: Kiwi juice

6 to 8pm: Spinach apple juice

Friday

8 to 9 am: Green juice with pears

10:30 to 11am: Watermelon flush

1 to 2 pm: Grapefruit and cranberry juice

3 to 4pm: Carrot turmeric juice

5 to 6pm: Grapes, prunes and strawberry juice

6 to 8pm: Almond milk and berry smoothie

Saturday

8 to 9 am: Green detox juice

10:30 to 11am: Parsley purifier

1 to 2 pm: Green warrior protein smoothie

3 to 4pm: Carrot orange juice

5 to 6pm: Powerful antioxidant juice

6 to 8pm: Anti-aging citrus juice

Sunday

8 to 9 am: The green machine

10:30 to 11am: Strawberry citrus juice

1 to 2 pm: Green protein boost juice

3 to 4pm: Tomato and beetroot juice

5 to 6pm: Antioxidant boost juice

6 to 8pm: Spicy green apple juice

There is plenty of scope for personalization and customization when it comes to a juice cleanse. You can use the recipes that you like. However, your primary goal must be to add as many nutrients to your daily intake as possible. During the juice cleanse, you will essentially be drinking juices and nothing else. Therefore, it is essential that you support these juices with other calorie-free beverages like herbal teas, water, and other supplements. You can also concentrate on engaging in light exercise and relaxation to make the process easier. Apart from that, there are different techniques you can use to speed up your body's overall detox.

Chapter Eight:

Optimize Your Success - How to Get the Most Out of Your Cleanse

Tips to Make the Juice Cleanse Easier

Starting and following a juice cleanse can seem a little intimidating, considering the fact that you will essentially be drinking all your meals for seven days. A juice cleanse is a simple dietary protocol. Preparing yourself, scheduling the fast, and planning for it are three simple steps you cannot afford to overlook if you want to successfully complete the 7-day juice cleanse.

If you want to make the most of the juice cleanse and optimize the results you attain, then here are some tips that will come in handy.

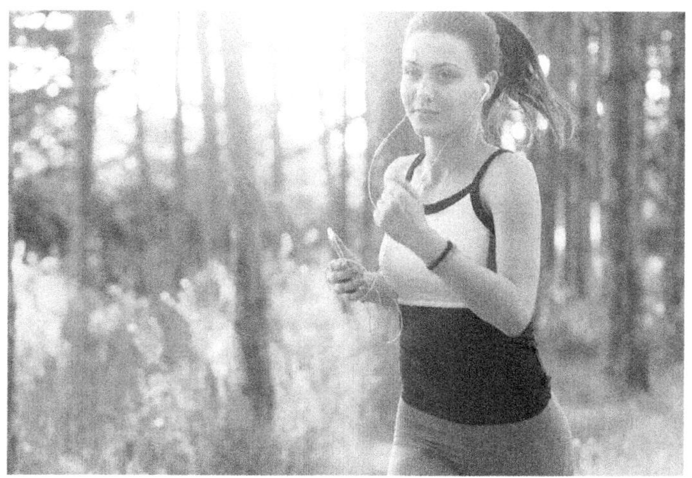

Light Exercise

You don't have to give up on exercising just because you are on the juice cleanse. Instead, try to tone down your workouts. Your body will require some time to get used to the new diet, and therefore, there will be fluctuations in your energy levels. If you exhaust yourself by engaging in high-intensity exercises, you run the risk of burning yourself out before even getting started with the cleanse. In fact, try to stick to light cardio exercises for the duration of this diet. After all, it is only for seven days, and after that, you can get back to your usual exercise routine.

Good Quality Sleep

Keep in mind that your body is not a tireless machine. It does need some time to recover, and its recovery time is usually longer during a juice cleanse. It is not just about sleeping but the quality of sleep you get that also matters. If you don't get sufficient sleep, it hinders your overall productivity in different aspects of your life. Sleep hygiene essentially consists of various practices and habits. You can use it to ensure that you get a good quality of sleep at night. There are a few sleep hygiene practices you can start following, like ensuring that you don't nap during the day, and if you nap, don't let it exceed 30 minutes. Start engaging in at least 10 minutes of aerobic exercise to promote the quality of sleep you get at night.

Avoid consuming substances like caffeine, alcohol, or nicotine late in the evening, or close to your bedtime. These stimulants tend to disrupt your sleep schedule. Ensure that your body gets sufficient exposure to sunlight during the day and darkness at night. It helps stabilize your circadian rhythm. Your circadian rhythm dictates your sleep cycle, and keeping it at an equilibrium is essential. You can create a regular relaxing bedtime routine, which will enable your body to recognize that it is time for bed. For instance, you can take a warm bath, listen to some soothing music, or even read a book before going to bed. Ensure that the sleep environment is pleasant and conducive to a good night's rest. The ideal temperature of the bedroom should be between 60 to 67°F. Turn off all bright lights, keep your cell phone away, turn off the TV, and your ability to sleep through the entire night will improve.

Understand Your Body

The primary idea of a juice cleanse to avoid consuming any solid food for seven days. However, if your body is telling you otherwise, then perhaps it is time to eat some light meals consisting of raw or steamed green vegetables or some egg whites. If you start feeling shaky, have any trouble concentrating, or feel lightheaded, then it is a sign that your body needs some form of solid food. Keep in mind that what might work for others doesn't necessarily have to work for you. Your body is quite different from that of others. Therefore, learn to understand what your body needs and cater to its needs.

Spa Day

Life is quite hectic, and giving yourself a break once in a while is the best thing you can do. So, take a day off and pamper yourself. Self-care is the best way to deal with the stresses of life. Regardless of whether you decide to head to the spa or indulge in some DIY at home, soaking in a luxurious bath or getting a massage will certainly help you feel better. When you feel better, your motivation levels will stay high, and it becomes easier to follow a diet.

Preparation

The more time your body has to prepare itself for the cleanse, the easier it will be to get through the cleanse. Usually, it is advised that you take at least a week to slowly ease your body into a juice cleanse. During this week, start increasing your intake of vegetables and fruits while gradually eliminating everything else. Believe it or not, your regular diet is addictive to your body. So, you must slowly wean yourself off all the foods you usually eat. Once you do this, sticking to a juice cleanse becomes quite easy. Also, learn to ease yourself out of the cleanse. Just because the cleanse ends doesn't mean your responsibility towards yourself does. Ease in and out of the cleanse to increase your chances of success.

Support System

Having a support system in place is a great way to keep up your motivation, especially on days when you feel low. Your support system can consist of your loved ones, family members, partner, friends, or anyone else. If you need resources, there are plenty of online forums or chat groups you can join to connect with others who are sailing in the same boat as you. Once you realize you aren't alone, it becomes easier to keep going.

Juice Fasting Journal Checklist

Start maintaining a journal to track the progress you make before, during, and after the fast. Maintain a journal about your juice fast journey so that sometime in the future, you can look back and see how much you have improved over time. With each fast, you have new information and insight into the things that do and don't work for you. This, in turn, gives you a chance to improve the overall fast experience. Ensure that a juice cleanse is not a once-in-a-lifetime event. Make it a part of your usual lifestyle. That said, don't do a 7-day juice cleanse twice a month. Or if you do want to attempt a long term juice cleanse, then maybe you can stick with the three-day variants. Regardless of what you decide to do, ensure that you listen to your body since it knows what it needs.

In the journal, make it a point to note down everything that you drink, the way you feel, your body's response, or any other detail you noticed while on a juice cleanse. You can also start jotting down your thoughts. Also, make a note of all the success, obstacles, and setbacks you might encounter. Here are some basic points you must include in the journal.

- How did I prepare myself for the juice cleanse?
- When did I start the juice cleanse?
- How many days do I want to follow the juice cleanse for?
- How is my overall health at present? (Mention any current health problems, if you have any)
- How much do I weigh?
- What juices do I include, and how much?
- Did I experience any reaction to the juices?
- How did I deal with any cravings or temptations?
- How do I feel during the juice cleanse?
- How are my energy levels?
- Am I able to get sufficient sleep?

- How did I end the juice cleanse?
- When did I end the juice cleanse?
- What did I do after the juice cleanse?
- How did I feel after the juice cleanse?

Once you answer all these questions, you will have a detailed account of all your juice cleanse experiences.

Mistakes to Avoid

A juice cleanse is a great way to detox your body and optimize your health. It is also an excellent way to flood your body with plenty of antioxidants, vitamins, and minerals. In this section, let us look at certain mistakes you must avoid if you want to make the most of a juice cleanse.

Mistake #1: Too much sugar

Juicing is a great way to pump nutrients into your body while optimizing its ability to absorb vitamins, enzymes, and minerals directly into the bloodstream. However, if you add too many fruits to the juice, you are essentially flooding your bloodstream with plenty of sugar. Fruits are a rich source of minerals, vitamins, and antioxidants, but they also contain a large source of fructose. If you want to avoid any unnecessary and frequent fluctuations in your blood sugar levels, it is important that you don't add too many fruits or sweet vegetables to your juices. If there are significant changes in your blood sugar levels, then it can make you feel tired and sluggish, defeating the purpose of a juice cleanse altogether.

The simplest way to avoid this is by following the 80:20 ratio for vegetables to fruits. If you follow this ratio while juicing, you can ensure that you don't flood your bloodstream with high doses of sugar.

Mistake #2: Not cold-pressed

Perhaps the best way to consume fresh fruits and vegetables in the form of juice is when it is cold press. A cold press uses a hydraulic press, which applies pressure for extracting the maximum amount of juice from vegetables and fruits. You can effectively prevent oxidation by cold pressing fruits and vegetables instead of squeezing or blending them. The cold press also helps ensure that the important enzymes and nutrients present in the ingredients stay in the juice. Therefore, before you start your juice cleanse, investing in a cold press juicer is a good idea.

Mistake #3: No immediate consumption

Another common mistake a lot of people make is that they don't consume the juice as soon as it is ready. If you want to make the most of juicing, then consume it while the juices are fresh. Juicing is not like a regular diet. You cannot make all the juices for the upcoming week and store it in the refrigerator. Whenever you make juice, consume it immediately, or it won't be as good. If you want to store it, then ensure that you consume it within 24 hours. Never store a juice for longer than 24 hours. It not only leads to the growth of mold and bacteria but also ruins the nutritional integrity of the juices you make.

Mistake #4: Caffeine intake

Before you start a juice cleanse, it is essential that you prepare your body for the cleanse. Therefore, you must remove different stimulants like nicotine, caffeine, and alcohol before you start juicing. Unless you do this, you cannot make the most of the benefits it offers. All the juices you consume during a cleanse will give your body all the energy it requires to keep going. Therefore, you no longer need to rely on your morning cup of coffee to wake you up. Instead, grab a fresh juice, and you will feel better. A common mistake a lot of people make while juicing is that they don't limit or avoid the consumption of alcohol, nicotine, or caffeine. All these substances will wreak havoc on your body. If you want to make the most of the cleanse, then avoid these stimulants.

Mistake #5: Insufficient hydration

During a cleanse, it is quite important that you keep your body thoroughly hydrated. About two-thirds of your body weight is made of water, and therefore it is important for the overall functioning of your body and mind. Dehydration can cause unpleasant symptoms like tiredness, headache, dizziness, and even extreme mood swings. Fruits and vegetables contain water, but you must drink at least eight glasses of water while on a juice cleanse. There is no alternative for sufficient hydration. If you want to flush out all the toxins from your body and regulate your hunger, then consuming water must be your priority.

Mistake #6: Drinking too quickly

Don't be in a hurry, and don't just gulp down the juice within a minute. Instead, take some time and try to work it around slowly before you swallow. By doing this, your body releases certain digestive enzymes that optimize the digestive process. It also helps to better absorb the different micronutrients present in the juice you consume. Also, if you made an effort to make the juice, then you can take a couple of minutes to savor the taste before guzzling it.

Mistake #7: Not drinking on an empty stomach

If you want to improve your body's ability to absorb all the micronutrients present in the juices and flush toxins out of your body, then you must drink juices on an empty stomach. If you keep consuming a regular diet, then it is not a juice cleanse. On a juice cleanse, all your meals and snacks will be in the form of juices, and nothing else. Unless you stick to this basic protocol, a juice cleanse will not work.

Mistake #8: No Pre-cleanse

A juice cleanse is not something that you can start without any preparation. You need to give your body a couple of days before the cleanse. It not only helps limit any of the side effects associated with the cleanse, bu also prepares you mentally for the cleanse. Physica preparation is as important as mental preparation when i comes to any diet. So, start increasing your intake of fruit and vegetables while reducing other foods, includin processed foods and sugars, at least a week before th juice cleanse.

By learning about these mistakes, you will be bette equipped to deal with a juice fast. Mistakes are certainl lessons, but at times, you can learn more from th mistakes others make. And you don't have to make then yourself.

Tips to Stay Motivated

When you start a new diet, you will be quite motivated t follow it. However, after a day or two, or maybe wher you start craving some food, this motivation starts fadin away. When the motivation goes away, the chances o following the diet also reduce drastically. To avoid all this it is important to stay motivated, and here are some tip you can use to do just that.

List Your Reasons

Before you start a juice cleanse, it is essential that you ar aware of your reasons for starting this diet. If you have n reason to start this diet, then it is quite likely that you' give up on it quickly. So, take some time, and think abou all the different reasons for wanting to do a juice fast

Whenever you notice that your motivation to follow the diet is reducing, just remind yourself of these reasons, and you will have the willpower to keep going.

Learn About Juice Cleanses

Carefully go through the information given in all the previous chapters up until now to learn more about juice cleanses. Unless you are aware of all the aspects of a juice cleanse, it becomes difficult to commit to it. Understand its purpose, the benefits it offers, and how it works in your body. Once you are aware of all this information, it becomes easier to prepare yourself mentally for the diet you wish to follow. Never start a diet unless you are mentally and physically prepared to stick to it until the very end.

Positive Mindset

Ensure that you keep a positive mindset about the diet. Don't expect any miraculous changes overnight. At least give this diet seven days if you want to see a positive change in your overall health and fitness. So, as long as you stick to the 7 days and follow the protocols of this diet carefully, you will notice an improvement in your energy levels, metabolism, and even lose weight along the way.

Inspiration

An effective way to motivate yourself to follow the diet is by reading through experiences of all those people who managed to attain their weight-loss goals through a juice cleanse. By reading success stories of others, it will give you the courage to keep going. It also helps when you understand that you are not alone, and there are others who are like you.

Planning

Ensure that you have planned the different juices you'll be consuming on each of the days while following a juice fast. Knowing what to juice, and when to drink will enable you to concentrate on your weight loss objectives. You can use the sample meal plan given in this book to get started.

Listen to Your Body

Always listen to your body whenever you make any dietary changes. While on a juice cleanse, your body is trying to detoxify and cleanse itself from within. This, in turn, might make you feel low on energy at times. Whenever you feel tired or restless, take a break and sleep. Whenever you feel hungry, drink some juice or water. Your body knows what it needs and, as long as you're paying attention to it, you can complete a juice cleanse successfully.

Get Creative

A common reason why a lot of people tend to give up on a juice cleanse is that they get bored with the juices they are drinking. Therefore, it is essential that you add some variety to your weekly meal plan. Include plenty of juices and mix various ingredients. As long as the ingredients can be mixed together, the sky's the limit. If you are running out of ideas, then start using the different recipes given in this book to get started. Once you get the hang of various flavor combinations, start experimenting. Regardless of what you do, ensure that you consume the juice immediately and don't allow it to rest for longer than 24 hours.

Fun and Relaxation

Ensure that your life is not just about work and stress. Take a break, relax, and do something you enjoy. When you are surrounded by people you love or are doing things you enjoy, your stress levels will reduce. Also, it helps improve your motivation to stick to the juice cleanse. There is no time like the present to learn a new hobby, read a good book, or even watch a movie. Spend some time with yourself and do things that you enjoy.

Visualization

A simple technique you can use to keep up your levels of motivation is visualization. Whenever you realize that you are running low on motivation, take a break from whatever you're doing. Now, it is time to concentrate on the goals you wish to attain by following the juice cleanse. Close your eyes, and visualize how wonderful you will feel once you attain your weight loss goals. Hold onto that feeling, and it will give you the motivation to keep going.

By following the simple tips discussed in this section, you

can ensure that your motivation levels stay high while following a juice cleanse.

It is important that you thoroughly plan the juice cleanse. Take some time out of your schedule and concentrate on different things that will enable you to make the most of the juice cleanse. Once your body and mind are thoroughly propagated, it becomes easier to start eliminating some foods before you start the cleanse. By doing this, the chances of sticking with it will increase, and the chances of experiencing withdrawal symptoms will reduce. Also, make it a point to consume organic, local, and seasonal ingredients. During this process, ensure that you get sufficient sleep, and pay close attention to the way you feel. It is a good idea to maintain a juice cleanse journal, or a weight loss journal. You can use this journal to even refine any of the recipes you use, and it will come in handy the next time you decide to follow a juice cleanse.

Chapter Nine:

Green Juice Recipes

All the recipes in this chapter are perfect for weight loss and made from low calorie ingredients.

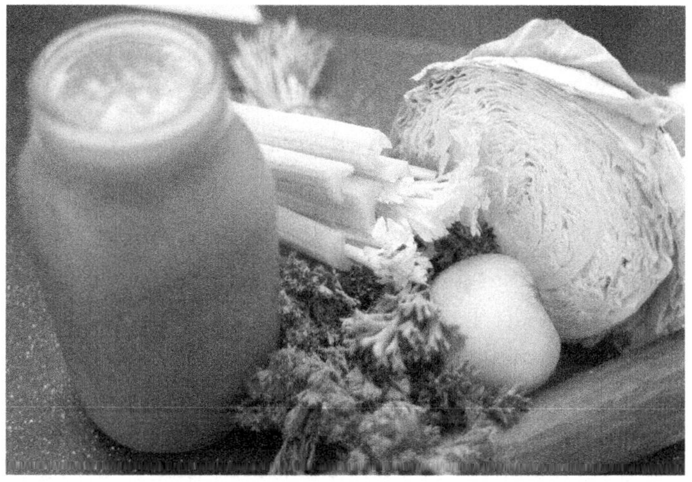

Green Detox Juice

Serves: 2

Ingredients:

- 4 green apples
- 2 cucumbers
- 1 lemon
- 2 sprigs mint
- 6 celery ribs
- 16 kale leaves
- 2 inches fresh ginger

Directions:

1. First, wash all the fruits and vegetables. Core the apples. Peel the lemon and cut it into 2 halves. Cut the celery into 1 inch pieces. Trim the cucumbers. Peel if desired.
2. Remove the hard stem and ribs from the kale. Tear the kale leaves.
3. Peel the ginger and cut it into slices. Chop the mint leaves.
4. Cut the apples and cucumbers into chunks (i should go into the feeder tube of the juicer easily)
5. Juice together the apples, lemon, ginger, mint celery, kale, and cucumber in the juicer. Put them into the juicer in the same order as is mentioned Apple goes in first, followed by lemon, ginger, etc
6. Pour into 2 glasses. Serve with crushed ice.

The Green Machine

Serves: 2

Ingredients:

- 2 cups packed baby spinach
- 2 large chard leaves
- 2 cups chopped, packed parsley
- 2 cups packed Romaine lettuce
- 2 cups baby kale leaves
- 2 stalks celery
- 2-inch fresh ginger
- 2 cucumbers
- 2 apples
- 2 cucumbers
- 4 tablespoons fresh lime juice (optional)
- 2 cups of coconut water

Directions:

1. Rinse all the greens well. Discard the hard stems and ribs, if any.
2. Rinse the cucumbers, ginger, and apples. Trim the cucumbers. Core the apples. Cut cucumber and apples into chunks that can slide easily into the feeder tube of the juicer.
3. Squeeze out juice from limes (if using lime juice) and measure out 4 tablespoons of lime juice. Use less lemon juice if you do not like the lemony taste. Set aside.
4. Add apples, ginger, greens, and cucumber, in the order mentioned, into the juicer and extract the

juice.

5. Take 2 tall glasses and divide the freshly extracted juice among the glasses.
6. Add 2 tablespoons of lime juice into each glass.
7. Add a cup of coconut water into each of the glasses. Stir until well combined.
8. Add ice if desired and serve right away.

Natural Energy Green Juice

Serves: 2 – 3

Ingredients:

- 3 cups coconut water
- 6 stalks celery
- 2 cups kale
- 4 cups spinach
- 2 bananas
- 2 cups of ice cubes
- 1 – 2 tablespoons ground cinnamon

Directions:

1. Discard hard stems from kale and spinach. Rinse well. Tear into smaller pieces and measure out. Slice the celery and bananas.
2. Add kale, spinach, celery, banana, cinnamon, ice cubes and coconut water into a blender.

3. Blend for 40 – 50 seconds or until very smooth.
4. Pour into 2 – 3 tall glasses and serve.

Electric Green Juice

Serves: 2

Ingredients:

- 2 cucumbers
- 2 cups spinach
- 2 cups parsley
- 4 green apples
- 2 cucumbers
- 4 inches fresh turmeric
- 4 beets
- Greens of 4 beets
- Juice of a lime

Directions:

1. Core the apples and cut into chunks. Wash all the greens and other vegetables.
2. Chop the beets and cucumber into chunks. Juice the lime.
3. Peel the turmeric and cut into slices.
4. Juice together all the ingredients in a juicer.
5. Pour into 2 glasses. Add lime juice and stir.

Green Juice with Pears

Serves: 3 – 4

Ingredients:

- 1 cup fresh parsley
- 1 lemon
- 12 large stalks celery
- 6 cups spinach
- 4 medium pears
- Ice cubes, as required

Directions:

1. Wash all the greens, pears, and lemon.
2. Peel the lemon. Chop the spinach, parsley, and celery. Core the pears and cut into wedges.
3. Add a few pear wedges into the juicer. Next, add in the greens and lemon.
4. Finally, add the remaining pears and extract the juice.
5. Divide into glasses. Add ice cubes and serve.

Chapter Ten:

Beet Juice Recipes

The recipes in this chapter are primarily made of beetroot, along with other healthy ingredients. Beetroot is high in fiber, potassium, iron, folates, and vitamin C. It is suitable for improving stamina, increasing blood flow, and lowering blood pressure.

Ginger-Beet Juice

Serves: 3 – 4

Ingredients:

- 2 oranges
- 2 apples
- 2 large beets
- Leaves of the beets
- 6 kale leaves
- 2 carrots
- 2-inch piece of fresh ginger

Directions:

1. Rinse all the fruits and vegetables. Cut the beets

and apples into wedges. Peel and slice the ginger.

2. Discard hard stems and ribs from the kale and beets. Tear into pieces. Peel oranges and separate into segments.
3. First, add oranges into the juicer followed by kale and apple. Next goes the beets, beet greens, and ginger. Last is the carrot.
4. Pour into glasses and serve with crushed ice.

Beetroot Juice

Serves: 2

Ingredients:

- 4 beets
- 6 stalks celery
- 1 cup fresh mint leaves
- 2 cucumbers
- 2 apples

Directions:

1. Wash all the vegetables and mint leaves. Trim the beets and cucumbers and cut them into chunks.
2. Core the apples and cut into chunks. Cut the celery into slices.
3. Add apples, mint, celery, cucumber, and beets into the juicer. Extract the juice and pour it into glasses.

4. Add ice and serve.

Tomato and Beetroot Juice

Serves: 2

Ingredients:

- 4 – 5 beets
- 6 tablespoons lime juice
- 4 – 5 tomatoes
- 1 cup mint leaves

Directions:

1. Trim the beets and cut them into wedges.
2. Chop the tomatoes into pieces.
3. Add beets, lime juice, tomatoes, and mint leaves into a blender and blend until smooth.
4. Pour into 2 glasses and serve.

Beet, Apple and Blackberry Juice

Serves: 2

Ingredients:

- 1 pound blackberries
- 6 medium beets
- 1-inch ginger

- 5 – 6 apples

Directions:

1. Rinse all the vegetables and fruits. Peel the apples if desired. Core the apples and cut into wedges.
2. Trim the beets and cut them into wedges. Peel and slice the ginger.
3. Juice together the apples and beets in a juicer.
4. Add blackberries, beets, and ginger into a blender. Pour the juice into the blender.
5. Blend for 30 – 40 seconds or until smooth.
6. Pour into glasses and serve with crushed ice.

Beet Treat

Serves: 2

Ingredients:

- 4 beets
- 6 carrots
- 2 oranges
- 2 cups spinach
- ¼ red cabbage
- Juice of a lemon
- 1 cup fresh pineapple chunks

Directions:

1. Wash all the fruits and vegetables.
2. Peel the beets and carrots and chop into small pieces. Chop the red cabbage as well.
3. Peel the oranges and discard the seeds. Remove the membranes on the orange segments as well.
4. Add all the fruits and vegetables into a blender and blend until smooth.
5. Pour into 2 tall glasses. Serve with crushed ice if desired.

Beet and Ginger Juice

Serves: 2

Ingredients:

- 2 large beets
- 1 bunch spinach
- 2 carrots
- 2 inches fresh ginger
- 2 apples

Directions:

1. Wash the vegetables and apples.
2. Trim and chop the beets and carrots into bite-size pieces.
3. Core the apple and cut into bite-size pieces.
4. Chop spinach into bite-size pieces.

5. Add apples into the juicer followed by spinach, ginger, beets, and carrots.
6. Pour into glasses and serve with crushed ice.

Chapter Eleven:

Carrot Juice Recipes

Carrots are one of the best antioxidant sources, which makes them great for a cleanse. They are high in beta carotenes, potassium, fiber, vitamin A and K and have cancer-fighting properties.

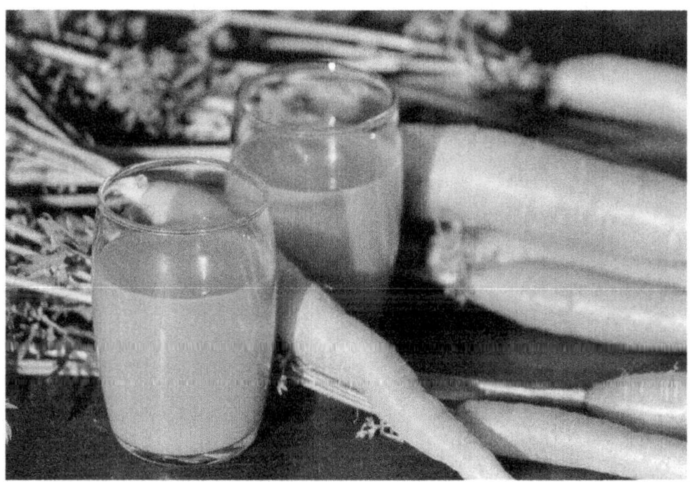

Mellow Mater Juice

Serves: 2-3

Ingredients:

- 4 medium tomatoes
- 2 large handfuls parsley or cilantro
- 2 large handfuls basil
- 4 carrots
- 2 cucumbers or zucchini
- 8 stalks celery
- 4 romaine lettuce leaves or cabbage leaves
- ½ lemon

Directions:

1. Rinse the chosen greens and all the vegetables.
2. Chop the tomatoes, carrots, celery, and cucumber or zucchini.
3. Add tomatoes, greens, carrots, cucumber, celery, and lettuce into the juicer.
4. Extract the juice and pour it into glasses.
5. Serve immediately.

Tropical Carrot Apple Juice

Serves: 2

Ingredients:

- 2 large apples
- 8 medium carrots
- 2 cups fresh pineapple chunks
- 2 inches fresh ginger
- 1 cup chopped papaya
- 1 kiwifruit

Directions:

1. Core the apples. Trim and chop the carrots. Peel and slice the ginger.
2. Juice together the apples, carrots, and ginger in a juicer and pour it into a blender.
3. Peel and chop the kiwifruit and add it into the juicer along with pineapple and papaya.
4. Blend until smooth. Add some ice cubes if desired and serve.

Carrot Turmeric Juice

Serves: 2

Ingredients:

- 10 medium carrots
- 2 inches fresh ginger
- 2 inches fresh turmeric
- 1 tablespoon honey
- Juice of a lemon

Directions:

1. Peel and slice the ginger and turmeric.
2. Trim the ends of the carrots. Cut into bite-size pieces.
3. Add some of the carrots into the juicer, followed by turmeric and ginger. Extract the juice.
4. Add remaining carrots and extract juice.
5. Pour into glasses. Add lemon juice and honey and stir.
6. Drink right away.

Skin Purifying Carrot Juice

Serves: 2

Ingredients:

- 10 medium carrots
- 2 handfuls spinach
- Juice of 2 lemons
- 8 kale leaves
- 2 cucumbers

Directions:

1. Rinse all the greens and vegetables.
2. Discard the hard stems and ribs of the kale and hard stems of spinach. Tear the greens.
3. Cut off the ends of the cucumbers and carrots and cut them into bite-size chunks.
4. Juice together the cucumbers, greens, and carrots in the juicer, in the same order as mentioned.
5. Divide into 2 glasses. Add lemon juice and stir.
6. Serve with crushed ice if desired.

Carrot Orange Juice

Serves: 2 – 3

Ingredients:

- 2 medium yellow tomatoes
- 2 apples
- 2 oranges
- 8 large carrots

Directions:

1. Wash the vegetables and fruits. Core the apples and peel the oranges.
2. Separate the segments of the oranges. Cut the tomatoes and apples into wedges.
3. Place the tomatoes into the juicer followed by oranges and apples and finally, the carrots.
4. Extract the juice and pour it into glasses.
5. Add some crushed ice if desired and serve right away.

Carrot Ginger Juice

Serves: 2

Ingredients:

- 12 medium carrots
- 4 inches ginger
- 2 oranges
- 1/8 teaspoon cayenne pepper
- 1 inch fresh turmeric

Directions:

1. Rinse the carrots, ginger, oranges, and turmeric.
2. Trim the ends of the carrots and cut them into bite-size pieces.
3. Peel the ginger, oranges, and turmeric. Slice the ginger. Separate the oranges into segments.
4. Juice together the turmeric, ginger, oranges and carrots, in the order mentioned.

Add cayenne pepper, stir, and serve.

Chapter Twelve:

Protein Juices

A protein juice cleanse brightens skin, helps reduce bloating, burns fat, and builds muscle mass in addition to being high in antioxidants.

Green Protein Boost Juice

Serves: 2

Ingredients:

- 16 Tuscan cabbage leaves
- 4 Swiss chard leaves with stems
- 10.5 ounces spinach
- 2 cups chopped pineapple
- 2 cucumbers
- Ice cubes, as required
- 2 scoops protein powder of your choice

Directions:

1. Rinse all the greens and cucumber. Trim and chop the cucumbers. Chop the Tuscan cabbage spinach, and Swiss chard.

2. Add cucumber into the juicer. Alternately add pineapple and greens (a little pineapple, a little greens and repeat this) into the juicer and extract the juice.
3. Pour the juice into a blender. Add protein powder and ice cubes and blend until smooth.
4. Pour into 2 glasses and serve.

Protein Powerhouse Green Juice

Serves: 2

Ingredients:

- 2 Granny Smith apples
- Juice of a lemon
- 2 inches fresh ginger
- 2 scoops pea protein powder
- 1 cucumber
- 2 stalks celery
- A large handful spinach
- 1 cup of water
- Ice cubes, as required

Directions:

1. Wash the vegetables and apples.
2. Core the apples. Trim the ends of the cucumber. Chop cucumber, apples, and celery into bite-size pieces. Add it into a blender.

3. Peel and slice the ginger and add it to the blender. Also, add water, ice cubes, lemon juice, spinach, and pea protein.
4. Blend for 30 – 40 seconds or until smooth.

Green Sprouts Juice

Serves: 6 – 8

Ingredients:

- 2 cups freshly brewed green tea, cooled
- 2 cups fresh alfalfa sprouts
- 2 cups fresh soybeans (edamame)
- 2 cups fresh wheat sprouts or wheatgrass
- 2 tablespoons pumpkin seeds
- 2 teaspoons chlorophyll
- 4- 5 cups of water

Directions:

1. Rinse soybeans, alfalfa sprouts, and wheatgrass. Chop the wheatgrass and soybeans if required and add them into a blender.
2. Add alfalfa sprouts, pumpkin seeds, chlorophyll, and green tea and blend until smooth.
3. Add water while blending if required. Pour into a jug without straining. Dilute with water.
4. It is best consumed on an empty stomach somewhere between 10 am – 2 pm. Drink the

juice very slowly. Once you drink the juice, it is best not to consume anything for 30 minutes.

Tomato and Alfalfa Juice

Serves: 2

Ingredients:

- 8 small tomatoes
- 2 tablespoons sunflower seeds
- ¼ teaspoon of sea salt
- 2 cups alfalfa (sprouted or plant)
- 2 sprigs parsley
- 1 teaspoon lemon juice

Directions:

1. Rinse the tomatoes and greens.
2. Cut the tomatoes into 2 halves.
3. Add tomatoes, sunflower seeds, salt, alfalfa, parsley, and lemon juice into a blender and blend until smooth.
4. Pour into glasses without straining.
5. This juice is to be sipped slowly in the evenings.

Almond Milk and Berry Smoothie

Serves: 4

Ingredients:

- ½ frozen strawberries
- ½ frozen blueberries
- 1 banana
- 4 cups vanilla almond milk, unsweetened, chilled
- ½ cup chopped fresh mango

Directions:

1. Peel and slice the banana.
2. Add berries, banana, mango, and almond milk into a blender and blend until smooth.
3. Pour into glasses and serve.

Green Warrior Protein Smoothie

Serves: 1 – 2

Ingredients:

- ½ pink grapefruit
- ½ large sweet apple
- 2 small celery stalks
- ¼ cup frozen mango chunks
- ¾ teaspoon virgin coconut oil (optional)
- 2 – 3 leaves Tuscan kale or ½ cup baby spinach

- 1 small cucumber
- 2 – 3 tablespoons hemp hearts
- A handful of fresh mint leaves
- Ice cubes, as required
- Water, as required

Directions:

1. Peel the grapefruit and separate into segments. Core the apple and trim the ends of the cucumber. Peel the cucumber if desired. Slice the celery stalks.
2. Pass the grapefruit through the juicer and extract the juice. Pour into a blender.
3. Add apple, celery, mango, kale, cucumber, coconut oil, ice, mint, hemp seeds, and a little water into the blender.
4. Blend for 40 – 50 seconds or until smooth.
5. Pour into glasses and serve.

Chapter Thirteen:

Anti-inflammatory Juice Recipes

As the name suggests, recipes in this chapter are perfec for an anti-inflammatory cleanse. The ingredients hel fight cancer, reduce pain and inflammation, and reduc bloating.

Pineapple, Turmeric, Cucumber, and Cinnamon Juice

Serves: 3

Ingredients:

- 1 cucumber, chopped
- 3 cups chopped fresh pineapple
- ½ tablespoon ground cinnamon
- 7 – 8 pieces fresh turmeric (3 inches each)

Directions:

1. Rinse the cucumber and turmeric. Peel and cut into pieces.
2. Add pineapple, cucumber, turmeric, and cinnamon into a blender.
3. Blend for 30 – 40 seconds or until smooth.
4. Divide into 3 glasses and serve.

Kale, Grape, Ginger and Lemon Juice

Serves: 2

Ingredients:

- 2 bunches kale
- 2 inches fresh ginger
- 2 cups grapes
- Juice of a lemon

Directions:

1. Rinse kale, grapes, and ginger thoroughly. Discard the tough stems and ribs of kale. Tear the leaves.
2. Add kale, ginger, and grapes into a blender and blend until smooth.
3. Strain if desired, and pour into glasses.
4. Add lemon juice and stir well. Add ice if desired and serve.

Anti-Inflammatory Tonic

Serves: 2

Ingredients:

- 8 carrots
- 2 oranges
- 6 stalks celery
- 2 inches fresh turmeric
- 1-inch fresh ginger
- Juice of a lemon

Directions:

1. Wash the fruits and vegetables thoroughly. Trim the carrots and cut into chunks that can enter the feeder tube of the juicer quickly.
2. Peel the oranges and separate into segments.
3. Peel the turmeric and ginger and cut into slices.
4. Place the oranges in the juicer, followed by turmeric and ginger.
5. Next, add in the celery and finally the carrots. Pour the juice into glasses.
6. Stir in lemon juice.

Anti-inflammatory Green Juice

Serves: 1 – 2 cups

Ingredients:

- 1.5 ounces fresh spinach

- 1-ounce flat-leaf parsley
- 1-inch fresh ginger
- 1 large apple
- Stevia drops to taste (optional)
- 1 large cucumber
- 1 teaspoon lemon juice

Directions:

1. Rinse the greens, apple, and cucumber. Core the apple and cut into wedges.
2. Peel and chop the cucumber into bite-size chunks.
3. First, add a little cucumber into the juicer, followed by a little of the greens. Next, add ginger and a small apple.
4. Add remaining cucumber, greens, and apples, in the same order as mentioned.
5. Pour into glasses. Add stevia drops if desired and serve right away.

Anti-inflammatory Vegetable Juice

Serves: 2

Ingredients:

- 2 broccoli heads
- 2 green apples
- 2 carrots

- 2 small cucumbers
- ½ cup Romaine lettuce
- 2 stalks celery
- Juice of ½ lime

Directions:

1. Wash the vegetables and fruits thoroughly. Core the apple and cut into chunks. It should slide easily into the feeder tube of the juicer.
2. Similarly, trim the carrots and cucumber and cut into chunks.
3. Cut the broccoli into small florets. Tear the lettuce and measure out ½ packed cup of lettuce. Slice the celery stalks.
4. Squeeze the juice from the lime.
5. Place the apples in the juicer followed by lettuce, celery, broccoli, carrots, and cucumbers.
6. Pour into glasses. Add lime juice and stir.
7. Serve right away.

Watermelon, Basil and Lime Juice

Serves: 4

Ingredients:

- 1 large watermelon
- Juice of a lime

- 1 cup fresh basil leaves, loosely packed

Directions:

1. Rinse the watermelon and basil.
2. Remove the rind of the watermelon and cut it into bite-size chunks. Discard the seeds.
3. Add watermelon, basil, and lime juice into a blender and blend until smooth.
4. Pour into glasses and serve.

Pineapple and Apple Juice

Serves: 4

Ingredients:

- 8 stalks celery
- 1 pineapple
- 4 handfuls fresh spinach
- 2 inches ginger
- 1 cucumber
- 1 green apple
- 2 lemons

Directions:

1. Wash all the ingredients.
2. Slice celery. Peel the lemons. Peel the pineapple and ginger. Cut pineapple into bite-size pieces. Slice the ginger.

3. Add celery, pineapple, spinach, ginger, cucumber, lemon, and apple into the blender, in the same order as is mentioned.

1.

Chapter Fourteen: Citrus Juice Recipes

The fresh burst of antioxidants and vitamin C from different citrus fruits is a great way to feel reenergized while giving your body essential nutrients.

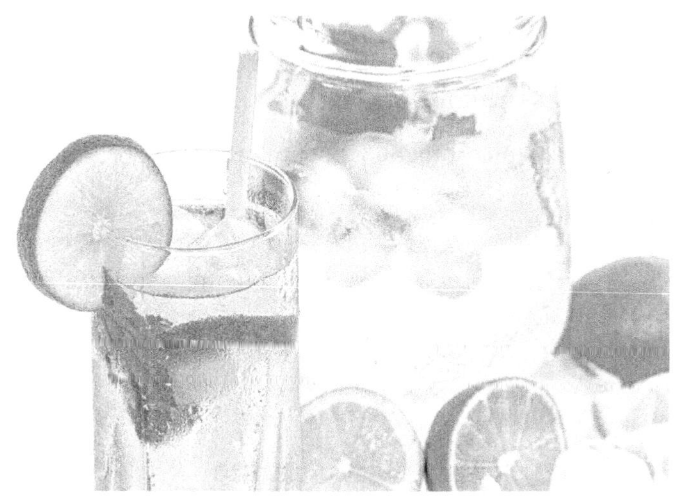

Grapefruit and Cranberry Juice

Serves: 2

Ingredients:

- 1 pink grapefruit
- ½ cup pure cranberry juice
- 2 small cucumbers
- Juice of ½ lime
- 1-inch fresh ginger (optional)
- 1 apple

Directions:

1. Wash the fruits and cucumbers. Cut the grapefruit into 2 halves horizontally. Juice the grapefruit in a citrus juicer.
2. Core the apple and cut into wedges. Peel the cucumber and cut into bite-size pieces.
3. Juice together cucumbers, ginger, and apple in a juicer.
4. Pour into 2 glasses. Add ¼ cup cranberry juice into each glass. Add lime juice and stir.
5. Serve right away. Keeping it for later will make it very bitter.

Anti-Aging Citrus Juice

Serves: 2

Ingredients:

- 6 – 7 mandarin oranges
- 1 grapefruit
- ½ lime
- 1 lemon
- 4 oranges

Directions:

1. Wash all the citrus fruits. Cut them into 2 halves horizontally.
2. Squeeze the juice of all the citrus fruits using a citrus juicer.
3. Stir well and pour into glasses.
4. Add ice and serve.

Strawberry Citrus Juice

Serves: 2

Ingredients:

- 1 grapefruit
- 2 navel oranges
- Juice of ½ lime
- 12 large strawberries

Directions:

1. Wash the fruits. Cut the oranges and grapefruit into 2 halves horizontally.
2. Squeeze the juice of oranges and grapefruit using the citrus juicer.
3. Pour into a blender. Add lime juice and strawberries into the blender and blend until smooth.
4. Serve immediately.

Spinach Apple Juice

Serves: 4

Ingredients:

- 1 bunch spinach
- 2 grapefruit
- 2 inches fresh ginger
- 4 green apples
- 2 cups fresh mint leaves
- 4 stalks celery
- Ice cubes, as required

Directions:

1. Rinse the fruits and vegetables.
2. Core the apples and cut into wedges. Peel the grapefruits. Separate into segments.
3. Slice the celery. Chop spinach into bite-size pieces.
4. Add grapefruit, greens, celery, ginger, and apples into the juicer. Extract the juice and pour it into glasses.
5. Serve with ice.

Chapter Fifteen: Colon Cleanse Juices

A colon cleanse improves your digestive system, helps in maintaining bowel movements, increases absorption of nutrition, weight loss, energy, and stamina, and reduce the risk of certain cancers.

Colon Cleanse Juice with Spinach and Apple

Serves: 1

Ingredients:

- 6 green apples
- 2 cups flat-leaf parsley
- 2 handfuls spinach

Directions:

1. Core and chop the apples.
2. Add apples, parsley, and spinach into a blender and blend until smooth. Add a little water whil

mixing.

3. Pour into glasses and serve.

Vegetable Juice

Serves: 2

Ingredients:

- 1 grapefruit
- 4 stalks celery
- 2 lemons
- 1 cucumber
- 2 apples
- 6 radishes with leaves
- 2 inches ginger

Directions:

1. Rinse all the vegetables and apples. Use only the tender leaves of the radish. Chop radishes.
2. Peel the grapefruit and lemons. Slice the celery.
3. Cut the apples. Peel and chop the cucumber.
4. Juice together the fruits and vegetables in the juicer.
5. Pour into glasses and serve with crushed ice.

Green Herbal Cleaner

Serves: 2

Ingredients:

- 6 stalks celery with leaves
- 2 handfuls parsley
- 4 handfuls spinach
- 2 cucumbers
- 2 carrots
- Juice of a lime
- 2 teaspoons linseed oil

Directions:

Wash all the greens, carrots, and cucumber with water.

Peel the cucumbers and cut them into pieces. Chop the parsley, spinach, carrots, and celery.

First, add cucumber into the juicer followed by spinach and parsley. Next goes in the celery and carrots. Add lime juice to the juice and stir well.

Pour into glasses. Add a teaspoon of oil to each glass and serve.

Colon Cleansing Carrot and Apple Juice

Serves: 2

Ingredients:

- 15 – 16 carrots
- 2 apples
- 2 large handfuls celery with leaves
- 2 large handfuls parsley

Directions:

1. Rinse the carrots, apples, and greens.
2. Trim the carrots and cut into chunks that can enter the feeder tube of the juicer quickly.
3. Chop the celery and parsley. Core the apples and cut into wedges.
4. Juice together the apples, greens, and carrots in the same order as mentioned.
5. Pour into glasses and serve right away.

Chapter Sixteen:

Heart Healthy Juice Recipes

Pear Cucumber Juice

Serves: 2

Ingredients:

- 10 – 12 leaves Tuscan kale
- 1 cucumber
- 2 pears
- 6 stalks celery
- 1 lemon

Directions:

1. Rinse the kale, cucumber, celery, lemon, and pears.
2. Core the pears. Trim the cucumber. Chop the cucumber and pears into chunks.
3. Slice the celery and peel the lemon.
4. Add pears and lemon into the juicer. Next, add celery, kale, and cucumber.
5. Pour into glasses and serve with crushed ice.

The Cholesterol Fighter

Serves: 2

Ingredients:

- 4 – 6 Swiss chard leaves
- 2 medium-size heads Romaine lettuce
- 2 inches fresh ginger
- 2 large cucumbers
- 2 medium-size Fuji apples
- 2 navel oranges

Directions:

1. Discard hard stems of chard leaves. Tear the leaves into smaller pieces. Tear the leaves of the lettuce as well.
2. Peel and slice ginger. Core the apples. Peel the cucumber. Chop apples and cucumber into bite-size pieces.
3. Peel the orange (but do not remove the pith) and separate it into segments
4. Juice together the ingredients, alternating apple, and cucumber with greens and orange.
5. Pour into glasses. Serve with crushed ice.

Spicy Green Apple Juice

Serves: 2

Ingredients:

- 4 green apples
- 4 capsicums
- 6 stalks celery
- Juice of a lemon

Directions:

1. Rinse the vegetables and apples.
2. Core the apples and cut into wedges.
3. Chop the capsicum into 1-inch pieces. Chop the celery into slices.
4. Add apples, capsicum, and celery into the juicer. Once the juice is extracted, add lemon juice and stir.
5. Pour into glasses and serve.

Heart Healthy Spinach and Garlic Juice

Serves: 2

Ingredients:

- 2 handfuls spinach
- 8 carrots
- 4 cloves garlic
- 2 apples
- 1 bunch parsley

- 1-inch fresh ginger

Directions:

1. Rinse the greens, carrots, and apples. Peel and rinse the ginger. Slice the ginger.
2. Trim the carrots and cut them into pieces. Peel the garlic. Chop parsley and spinach.
3. Add apples into the juicer. Next, add the greens, garlic, and ginger. Finally, add the carrots. Once the ingredients are juiced, pour into glasses.
4. Serve right away.

Cucumber Cooler

Serves: 2

Ingredients:

- 8 carrots
- 2 cucumbers
- 2 Granny Smith apples
- 2 limes
- 6 stalks celery
- 2 leaves Romaine lettuce
- 3 – 4 cups broccoli florets
- 1 cup blueberries
- 2 teaspoons flaxseeds

Directions:

1. Rinse all the fruits and vegetables.
2. After trimming the carrots, cut them into pieces. Peel and chop cucumber into chunks.
3. Core and chop apples. Peel the limes. Slice celery and lettuce.
4. Juice together broccoli, lettuce, celery, limes, apples, cucumber, and carrots.
5. Pour into a blender. Add blueberries and flax seeds. Blend until smooth.
6. Pour into glasses and serve.

Chapter Sixteen:

Antioxidants Juice Recipes

An antioxidant cleanse helps reduce oxidative stress in the body, which in turn helps fight cancer, heart disease, arthritis, repairs tissue damage and increases immunity.

Antioxidant Boost Juice

Serves: 2

Ingredients:

- 4 mini cucumbers
- 3 kale leaves, with stem
- 1 ambrosia apple
- 1 inch fresh ginger
- 6 stalks celery

Directions:

1. Rinse all the vegetables and the apple.
2. Chop kale leaves as well as stems. Core and chop the apple. Slice the celery and ginger (after peeling).

3. Add kale into the juicer followed by ginger and cucumber. Next comes the apple, followed by celery.
4. Pour into glasses and serve with ice.

Powerful Antioxidant Juice

Serves: 2

Ingredients:

- 6 cups chopped Swiss chard
- 4 sprigs celery leaves
- 1 medium beet
- 8 sprigs mint
- 2 carrots
- 2 oranges
- 1/8 teaspoon rock salt (optional)
- Ice cubes, as required

Directions:

1. Rinse all the greens thoroughly.
2. Trim the carrots and cut them into pieces. Peel the oranges and beets and cut them into wedges.
3. Add carrots into the juicer. Next, add greens followed by oranges and beets.
4. Divide into glasses. Add ice cubes and rock salt and stir well.

5. Serve right away.

Grape Prunes and Strawberry Juice

Serves: 2 – 3

Ingredients:

- 2 cups grapes (the variety with seeds)
- 1 cup prunes
- 1 cup chopped strawberries
- 1 ½ cups water
- 2 tablespoons pumpkin seeds
- 2 tablespoons honey or to taste

Directions:

1. Measure all the fruits after rinsing well.
2. Cut the grapes into 2 halves. Do not discard the seeds as the seeds contain antioxidants.
3. Add all the fruits, water, and pumpkin seeds into a blender and blend until smooth.
4. Make sure not to strain the juice.
5. Pour into glasses. Add honey and stir.
6. Sip slowly and enjoy your juice.

Kiwi Juice

Serves: 2 – 3

Ingredients:

- 4 cups fresh, chopped pineapple
- 8 kiwis
- 4 inches fresh ginger
- 6 red apples
- 2 stalks celery
- 1 cup fresh mint leaves

Directions:

1. Wash all the fruits and greens.
2. Add apples into the juicer. Next, add the mint, ginger, and celery. Next goes in the kiwis and pineapple.
3. Once the juice is made, pour into glasses and serve immediately.

Chapter Seventeen:

Liver Cleanse Juices

Detox your liver and gallbladder using the different juice recipes given in this chapter. Keep your liver happy with various cleansing juices made of fresh herbs and vegetables.

The Liver Scrubber Juice

Serves: 2

Ingredients:

- 2 large apples
- 2 whole beets
- 2 stalks celery
- 6 beet green leaves
- 8 medium carrots
- 1-inch ginger

Directions:

1. Core the apples and cut into wedges. Trim the beets and cut them into wedges.

2. Tear the beet leaves, discarding the stems. Trim the carrots and cut them into bite-size pieces. Peel and slice the ginger. Slice the celery as well.
3. Juice together carrots, ginger, beet greens, celery, beets, and apples in the juicer.
4. Pour into glasses and serve with crushed ice.

Liver Cleansing Juice

Serves: 2

Ingredients:

- 4 stalks celery
- 4 medium carrots
- 2 inches fresh ginger
- 2 apples
- 4 medium cucumbers (optional)
- 1 bunch spinach
- 2 small beets
- 2 small lemons
- Stevia drops to taste
- ¾ teaspoon Livatrex drops

Directions:

1. Rinse all the vegetables and fruits.
2. Peel and slice the ginger and lemon.
3. Trim carrots and beets and cut into bite-size

chunks. Peel the cucumber and cut it into pieces. Core and slice apples into wedges.

4. Juice together carrots, greens, beets, ginger, and lemon. Next goes in the cucumber and apples.
5. Divide into 2 glasses. Add Stevia and Livatrex drops among the glasses and serve right away.

Dandelion Green Juice

Serves: 2

Ingredients:

- 3 handfuls dandelion greens
- 2 beets
- 2 cucumbers
- 2 apples
- 1 teaspoon turmeric powder
- 2 lemons

Directions:

1. Rinse dandelion greens, beets, cucumbers, lemons, and apples.
2. Core and chop apples. Peel and chop cucumbers. Scrub the beets and cut them into chunks.
3. Pass the beets, greens, cucumbers, lemons, and apples into the juicer and extract the juice.
4. Pour into glasses and drink immediately. This juice will be bitter in taste because of dandelions.

"Liver Purifier" Juice

Serves: 2

Ingredients:

- 1 beet
- 4 carrots
- 4 stalks chard
- 1 cucumber
- 6 stalks celery
- 2 handfuls dandelion roots
- Juice of a lemon

Directions:

1. Wash all the vegetables and dandelion roots.
2. Trim the carrots and beets and cut into bite-size pieces.
3. Chop celery and chard.
4. Juice together beets, carrots, dandelion roots, chard, celery, and cucumber in the juicer.
5. Divide into 2 glasses and serve.

Chapter Eighteen:

Kidney Cleanse Juice Recipes

All the recipes given in this chapter are the perfect home remedies to detox and flush your kidneys. These juices promote hydration and better absorption of nutrients while flushing out extra toxins from the body.

Kidney Detox Juice

Serves: 2

Ingredients:

- 8 cucumbers
- 8 stalks celery
- Juice of 2 limes

Directions:

1. Wash the celery and cucumbers.
2. Peel and chop cucumbers into bite-size pieces.

Cut celery into ½ inch pieces.

3. Juice together celery and cucumbers in the juicer.
4. This should make about 4 glasses of juice. Hav this 4 times during the day.

Kidney Cleanse Juice

Serves: 2

Ingredients:

- 4 stalks celery
- 8 medium cucumbers
- 2 apples
- 4 medium carrots
- 2 medium beets
- 2 oranges

Directions:

1. Trim the carrots and cut them into pieces. Pee the cucumber and cut into pieces.
2. Peel oranges and separate into segments.
3. Core and chop the apples into chunks. Cho carrots, beets, and celery into bite-size pieces.
4. Add celery and carrots into the juicer. Next, ad cucumbers, beets, and apples. Finally, ad oranges.
5. Divide the juice into glasses and serve right away.

Kidney Cleanse Juice

Serves: 2

Ingredients:

- ½ cup cranberries
- 2 dates or 1 tablespoon date paste or 1 tablespoon pure maple syrup
- Juice of a lemon
- 3 – 4 mint leaves
- 2 cups water, divided
- 1 red apple
- ½ tablespoon ground cardamom

Directions:

1. Place cranberries into a pot. Pour 1 ½ cups of water and place the pot over medium heat.
2. When it comes to a boil, remove from heat and let it cool to room temperature. Pour into a glass jar.
3. Add dates, lemon juice, and remaining water into a blender and blend until smooth.
4. Pour into the glass jar.
5. Rinse and core the apple. Cut into slices. Add apple slices, cardamom and mint leaves into the jar and mix well.
6. Serve.

Watermelon Flush

Serves: 2

Ingredients:

- 3 cups cubed, deseeded watermelon
- 1 teaspoon lemon juice or to taste
- 8 – 10 fresh basil leaves

Directions:

1. Add watermelon and basil into a blender and blend until smooth.
2. Add lemon juice and blend again.
3. Pour into glasses and serve.

Parsley Purifier

Serves: 2

Ingredients:

- 1 cup fresh parsley
- 2 carrots
- 4 celery ribs
- 2 cucumbers

Directions:

1. Wash the vegetables thoroughly.

2. Trim and chop carrots. Slice celery and parsley. Peel and chop cucumber.
3. Juice together carrots, celery, parsley, and cucumber, in the juicer.
4. Divide into glasses and serve.

Chapter Nineteen:

You've Finished Your Juice Cleanse... Now What?

How to End a Cleanse

As soon as the juice cleanse ends, give yourself a moment to rejoice your accomplishment. You have managed to stick to a juice cleanse for a week, and it is not a small feat. For each day that you follow the juice cleanse, you provide your body with all the nourishment it requires. You give your body a chance to cleanse itself from within while optimizing your overall health. Bask in this feeling and pat yourself on the back. Take a moment and think about how you feel immediately after the cleanse ends. Make a note of all that you have learned and the different tips you might want to use even after the cleanse. Just because the juice cleanse ends, it doesn't mean you are about to return to unhealthy patterns of eating. Keep in mind that you worked quite hard to break free of the vicious cycle of unhealthy food dependencies. Therefore, it is time to make a healthier and more sustainable dietary regimen for yourself.

What to Eat?

As soon as the juice cleanse ends, ensure that the day after it, you consume plenty of vegetables and fruits or nuts. The vegetables you eat must be either raw or lightly steamed. Don't go overboard and consume small meals. The diet you follow will be quite similar to the one you followed while preparing for the juice cleanse. It essentially means you must stay away from sugar, processed foods, gluten, wheat, coffee, alcohol, or any other dairy products. The next day, you can add more plant-based foods like brown rice, beans, or even quinoa. Likewise, you will keep adding all the foods you previously used to eat but will do so gradually. Here is a simple sample of how your diet must look for five days after a juice cleanse.

Day 1

You can consume fresh vegetables in the form of salads, steamed vegetables, vegetable soup, carrot sticks, or celery sticks. You can also consume fresh fruit and nuts. However, don't consume more than a handful of nuts. Add different spices and herbs to flavor the food you eat. Always opt for coconut or extra virgin olive oil to cook any of your meals.

Day 2

You can add some plant-based healthy and wholesome carbs to your diet like brown rice or quinoa. Don't forget to add fresh and steamed vegetables. Apart from that, you can introduce starchy vegetables like sweet potatoes. You can also add beans, legumes, fruits, and nuts. Once again, cook your meals using coconut oil or extra virgin olive oil. Don't forget to add various herbs and spices to flavor the food you consume.

Day 3

Now, you can add some dairy products to your diet, if you want to. Ideally, on the third day after a juice cleanse you can consume vegetables, fruits, nuts, beans, legumes, brown rice, quinoa, organic yogurt (unsweetened and unflavored), eggs, and small amounts of plant-based oils.

Day 4

From this day onward, you can slowly reintroduce meat, fish, and poultry, if you want to. The foods you can consume on the fourth day after a juice cleanse are vegetables, fruits, nuts, beans, legumes, brown rice, quinoa, organic yogurt (unsweetened and unflavored), eggs, tofu or edamame, animal protein (meat, fish, or chicken), and small amounts of plant-based oils.

Day 5

Once you have followed the dietary guidelines mentioned up until now, your body will be used to your usual diet. You can pretty much eat anything that you want. However, don't use it as an excuse to binge on unhealthy food and stay away from all these types of foods for a while. Ensure that you are consuming healthy and wholesome meals. If you want to make the most of the benefits you derived from a juice cleanse, it is essential that you stick to a healthy diet.

Reintroducing Foods

Usually, people tend to take a couple of days after a juice cleanse to identify the way the body reacts to certain foods. It does take a while, but it can provide significant insights about any reactions to some foods you might not have noticed otherwise. You can maintain a food journal while reintroducing food systematically. Notice if there are any changes in your cravings, energy, digestion, or any other symptoms whenever you reintroduce a specific food. It is ideal that you use a specific limit of a type of food and watch its quantity.

For instance, if you have introduced gluten on the first day in small amounts twice or thrice a day in the form of bread, pasta, etc., notice how your body reacts in the next 24-48 hours. Another category of food you must test for any food sensitivity is dairy. For instance, have a couple of pieces of cheese or a glass of milk and wait for 24 to 48 hours to notice any reactions.

If there is a specific food group that doesn't suit your body, there are still a couple of ways in which you can enjoy them. Perhaps you can try avoiding it altogether for a while or consume them in smaller quantities. There are certain food alternatives that you can still consume in the same amount. For instance, you can replace regular milk with lactose-free milk or beans with any variants that contain enzyme supplements. If you need any further guidance, always consult your primary care provider or a qualified nutritionist.

Activities

Give yourself and your body at least three days before you resume any vigorous or strenuous activities. Your body just went through a significant change during the juice cleanse. Therefore, give it some time to get used to the usual routine. You might feel a little tired after the diet, so take a break. Concentrate on consuming healthy, light, and wholesome meals. It is essential to add some form of physical exercise to your daily routine. However, it doesn't mean you resume high-intensity training exercises on the first day after the cleanse. Take three to five days before engaging in any physically tiring or strenuous activities.

Maintain a Journal

If weight loss is your priority, then it is important that you come up with a dietary regimen that enables you to maintain the weight you lost during the juice cleanse. The simplest way in which you can do this is by maintaining a weight loss journal. The first step is to decide all the different aspects of your life you wish to record. Regardless of all that you want to include, don't forget to include recordings of your daily food intake and drink consumption. In this section, let us look at some simple tips you can follow while maintaining a weight loss journal.

Keep track of all the nutrients you consume. Make a note of the portion size and the nutrition your body gets. Keep in mind that the portion size you consume could be quite different from the serving size mentioned in the nutritional facts labels on foods. There are plenty of websites and apps you can use to obtain nutrition data about calories, carbs, fiber, proteins, and fats present in specific ingredients.

Start making a note of all your mealtimes. Whenever you eat, record the time, and how long you take to consume a meal. This enables you to identify whether you are eating too quickly or too often. If you eat quickly, it often leads to overeating since your body doesn't get sufficient time to recognize when it is full. If you eat too often, it might be a sign that you are consuming empty calories that don't sate your hunger. If that's the case, then you will quickly end up regaining all the weight you lost during the juice cleanse. Apart from that, by consciously noting down the meal times, it enables you to regularize your meals.

Start recording your environment at mealtime. If you want some insight into the different factors which influence your eating habits, record when you eat, and what time. If you eat alone, do you sit in front of the laptop, or the television? Do you always sit down at the dining table for a meal, or do you stand in the kitchen and gobble up your meal quickly? Do you tend to overeat when you are with people you love? By answering these questions, you can start making changes to your eating schedule and pattern.

Learn to become conscious of your body's hunger cues. Before every meal, try to rate your hunger on a scale of one to 5, with one being not hungry and five being extremely hungry. By practicing this simple exercise, and mindfulness, you become aware of your hunger. Learn to eat only when you are hungry and not just because you are used to eating at a specific time.

The final step is to record your emotions whenever you eat. Did you eat in response to any strong emotions or stress? If yes, then it is a sign of emotional eating. It essentially means you must start regulating your emotions before you use food as a coping mechanism. Make a note of how you feel before and after every meal. After a while, you will understand the emotions that trigger your hunger. Once you identify the triggers, it becomes easier to regulate your emotions and manage your hunger. Keep in mind that there are plenty of coping strategies, and eating is not one of them.

By following the simple steps and tips discussed in this section, you can effectively regulate your hunger and become conscious of the food you consume. Keep in mind that a food journal is merely a tool for self-reflection. Don't judge or be ashamed of your eating habits. There is always scope for improvement. Unless you identify the problem, you cannot improve yourself.

Diet to Follow

Maintaining a healthy diet is vital, and one of the best diets one can follow is a Mediterranean diet. As the name suggests, this diet is based on eating patterns or the traditional cuisine of countries in the Mediterranean region. This diet is mostly rich in plant-based produce and olive oil. A Mediterranean diet encourages the intake of fresh vegetables, fresh fruits, whole grains, and seafood. It effectively restricts the consumption of red meat and dairy products. Unlike regular diets, the Mediterranean diet doesn't place any emphasis on counting calories. You no longer have to count every single calorie you consume. As long as you concentrate on consuming high-quality and nutrient-dense ingredients, that is all you need to do. The Mediterranean diet includes five essential food groups, which are vegetables, fruits, protein, grains, and limited amounts of dairy.

While following this diet, ensure that you consume at least 2 to 3 cups of vegetables daily. Try to avoid or limit your intake of red meats. Don't consume them more than twice or thrice a week, and instead, replace red meat with naturally healthy and fatty fish like salmon, trout, sardines, or anything else you can think of. The Mediterranean diet encourages the consumption of dairy products in limited amounts. Certain dairy products can be added to your meals, including Greek yogurt and cheese. You must eat plenty of fresh fruits while following the Mediterranean diet. Instead of consuming sugar-rich and nutrient lacking processed foods, replace them with fresh and seasonal fruits. The Mediterranean diet encourages the consumption of plenty of healthy fats. Use nut based butter and olive oil for cooking all your meals. There are no dietary restrictions about the consumption of grains. Stay away from processed flour and concentrate on consuming whole grains. As a rule of thumb, stay away from anything that looks like it was produced in a factory. Avoid unhealthy and processed foods rich in unhealthy fats, carbs, sugars, food colorings, and other additives. By reducing your intake of processed foods, your daily diet becomes healthy. It is one of the reasons why the

Mediterranean diet is the perfect diet after a juice cleanse Stick to this diet if you want to maintain your weight los and lead a healthier life.

Tips for Additional Weight Loss

In this section, let us look at certain tips you can use tc maintain your weight loss after a juice cleanse.

Hydration Matters

Regardless of whether you are on a juice cleanse or hav successfully completed it, hydration is a must. Your bod must be hydrated all the time. If not, be prepared to dea with some unpleasant side effects like mild headaches mood swings, and tiredness. Whenever you drink water, i helps your body flush out all the toxins. It will defeat th purpose of a cleanse if your body is back to square on after the cleanse. Drinking water is also a great way t curb unhealthy cravings. Whenever you start cravin some unhealthy junk, drink a glass of water, give yoursel a couple of minutes, and go back to the task at hanc Ensure that you drink at least eight glasses of water daily.

Add Exercise

Don't forget to add some sort of physical activity to you daily routine if you want to maintain your weight los You don't necessarily have to go to the gym and exercis Even some light cardio like running, jogging, swimmin yoga, dancing, and biking help give your body a chance t burn the calories you consume. If you enjoy playing an outdoor sports, then you can do that, too. As long a there is some form of movement added to your daily routine, maintaining weight loss becomes more natural.

Healthier Food Choices

Don't be under the misconception that eating less is equivalent to losing weight. Yes, your body must stay in a calorie deficit for promoting weight loss, but it doesn't mean you eat less. Instead, learn to make healthier food choices. If you want to lose weight and maintain weight loss, a healthy diet is quite essential. Perhaps you could follow a Mediterranean diet as previously outlined.

Even if you don't follow a specific diet, ensure that you are consuming healthy and wholesome meals instead of eating junk food. For instance, your daily calorie intake must be between 1800 to 2500 calories. You can either eat a pint of ice cream and a burger in this calorie range or eat three healthy and wholesome meals. If weight loss is your priority, then binging on such unhealthy junk will lead to weight gain. Even if, by some miracle, you manage to stay in a calorie deficit, you are depriving your body of all the essential nutrients it requires to function optimally. So, don't do this, and learn to make healthier food choices.

Hidden Carbs

Learn to be wary of various hidden carbs. Markets these days are flooded with prepackaged foods that offer convenience, but come at a high cost. Carefully go through the list of ingredients before you make any purchase. Even the items that claim to be calorie-free, zero-calorie, or low calorie tend to contain some form of carbs or the other. If you notice any ingredient that you don't recognize, then avoid purchasing such a product. If you are careful, such carbs can quickly creep up on you, and increase your calorie intake. For instance, most of the sugar-free products in the market these days contain various artificial sweeteners in them.

Fats are Good

Stop fearing fats, since healthy fats are good for you. It is a popular misconception that fats are bad for your health. In fact, carbs and sugars are bad for your overall health. Instead, learn to add certain sources of healthy monounsaturated and omega-3 fatty acids to your daily meals. Stay away from all products that contain saturated fats, hydrogenated oils, and trans fats. Include healthy fats like avocados, naturally fatty fish (salmon, herring, sardines, trout), eggs, and extra virgin olive oil to your diet.

Track Your Progress

The simplest and quickest way to ensure that you are moving towards your weight loss, fitness, or health goals is by tracking the progress you make. Use the weight loss journal mentioned in the previous section to track your progress after the cleanse. You can also download an app to help you do this. There are plenty of paid and free applications available these days that can help you effectively track your calorie intake and meals you consume.

Plan Your Meals

Regardless of the diet, you wish to follow, always plan your meals ahead. By doing this, it not only reduces the stress of figuring out what your next meal will be but prevents the chances of bingeing on unhealthy foods. For instance, if you know there is a healthy meal waiting for you at home, the chances of eating out, or wanting to order takeout, will reduce. In the long run, it helps decrease your food budget, while making sure that you are eating healthy and wholesome meals. By planning your meals ahead, you can also quickly shop for the required groceries and stock your pantry with them. Once all the ingredients you need to cook are readily available, it becomes easier to prepare healthy meals.

Remove Temptations

When it comes to diets, out of sight and out of mind is the best way to go about it. If you are constantly surrounded by temptations, then the urge to straying away from a healthy diet increases. Therefore, it is time to clean your kitchen and pantry of all the unhealthy items that are usually tempting. So, it is time to say goodbye to cookies, chocolate, ice cream, chips, or any other junk food you can think of. When there are no temptations around you, then your mind will not start thinking about them. It is a simple technique of diverting your attention from undesirable thoughts toward something more desirable. Once you have removed all the unhealthy items, start replacing them with healthy alternatives.

Keep Yourself Busy

One of the best ways to get accustomed to a new diet is by keeping yourself busy. If you are occupied with work or indulging in any hobby you enjoy, then you will not have the time to think about eating. So, try to distract your mind as much as you can, at least during the initial couple of days. When you stop obsessing over what your next meal will be, the temptation to binge on unnecessary foods will also decrease. By keeping yourself thoroughly occupied with work, or any other activity, you can improve your overall productivity as well. So, whenever you start a new diet, ensure that you are busy, and your mind is distracted.

Probiotics

A juice cleanse helps detoxify your body from within while promoting your digestive system's ability to function optimally. To ensure that your digestive system does its job well, add some probiotics to your meals. Your gut is home to millions of bacteria known collectively as your gut microbiome. When this microbiome functions like it is supposed to, it helps maintain your digestive health. As with any other bacteria, even your gut microbiome requires some sustenance. The best nutrition you can offer them are probiotics. Different types of probiotics you can consume are yogurt, kombucha, and sauerkraut. Start eliminating pro-inflammatory foods like alcohol, weight, processed sugar, processed flour, and carbs while increasing the intake of anti-inflammatory foods. By doing this, you can ensure that your body's metabolism functions optimally.

Mindful Eating

We all tend to lead extremely busy and hectic lives these days. Mindful eating is a simple technique that enables you to make healthier food choices while making you conscious of your eating patterns. Whenever you eat, ensure that all your attention is directed towards the meal you're eating, and nothing else. Get rid of all distractions, especially electronic gadgets. So, stop sitting in front of the television, laptop, or smartphone while you eat. Instead, concentrate on the food you eat. Try to notice the different textures present and learn to savor every morsel you consume. Did you know that it takes your stomach 20 minutes to realize when it is full? When you slow down and thoroughly chew your food befor swallowing and don't just gobble it up in a hurry, i reduces the chances of overeating. Also, when yo thoroughly chew your food and swallow, it make digestion and absorption of that food quite easy.

To make the most of the benefits associated with a juic cleanse and for transitioning smoothly into your regula diet, it is important that you are mindful of the day following the cleanse. Before you start consuming an solid food, start reintroducing separate food item gradually. In the same way you eliminate certain foo groups before the juice cleanse, you must add them bac to your diet. Don't forget to incorporate the differen lessons you learned during the cleanse once the diet ends If you want to maintain weight loss, you need t concentrate on following a healthy dietary regimen an add some physical activity to your daily routine. B keeping these two simple tips in mind, you can make th most of a juice cleanse even after it ends.

Conclusion

In this book, you were given simple steps and strategies you can use to start and successfully end a seven-day juice cleanse. A juice cleanse is an effective way to lose weight, but that certainly isn't the only benefit it offers. A juice cleanse can improve your body's metabolism, detoxify it from within, and give you a much-needed energy boost. The cleansing powers of juicing are steadily gaining popularity and have taken the world of fitness by storm. If you are looking for ways to quickly shed those extra pounds and start a healthy new life, then this book has all the information you need.

By now, you will have undoubtedly realized how simple juicing is. You don't require any expensive or fancy ingredients, and you certainly don't have to spend hours in the kitchen to follow this diet. As long as your pantry is stocked with the necessary ingredients, you have nothing else to worry about. It barely takes a couple of minutes to whip up a nutritious, tasty, and filling juice. Sticking to a diet has never been this simple or easy to incorporate. The great thing about a juice cleanse is that regardless of how hectic your usual lifestyle is, you can follow this diet.

Learn to be patient with yourself while following this diet. If you stick to this diet for at least seven days, you will notice wonderful changes in your body. You will no longer have to count your calories because your calorie intake will reduce on a juice cleanse. All that you need to do is merely follow the simple protocols laid out by this diet and come up with a maintenance plan for sustaining the weight loss. As long as you consume healthy and wholesome meals while reducing the intake of unhealthy foods, you can improve your overall health. So, all that is left for you to do is get started with this wonderful diet. Take the first step towards a healthier life with a juice cleanse. I hope you found the book informative, and I hope that it helps you in your quest to get started on your juicing journey.

Thank you and all the best!

References

10 Innocent Signs That Your Body Is Flooded With Toxins. Retrieved https://brightside.me/inspiration-health/10-innocent-signs-that-your-body-is-flooded-with-toxins-722510/

A Step-By-Step Guide To Surviving Your First 3 Day Juice Cleanse — Pure Green Juice and Smoothies. (2016). Retrieved from https://www.puregreen.com/pure-green-magazine/surviving-a-3-day-juice-cleanse

Brown, M. (2019). Juicing: Good or Bad?. Retrieved from https://www.healthline.com/nutrition/juicing-good-or-bad#whole-fruits-and-veggies)

Calories during a Juice Cleanse - Yogic Way of Life. Retrieved from https://www.yogicwayoflife.com/calories-during-a-juice-cleanse/

Can I Juice Cleanse when I am pregnant or breastfeeding?. (2015). Retrieved from https://solcleanse.com/2015/06/01/juice-cleanse-pregnant-breastfeeding/

How To Do a Juice Cleanse | Project Juice. (2019). Retrieved from https://www.projectjuice.com/how-to-cleanse

Juice Cleanse To Lose Weight Fast | Juicing Diet Plan | CAN CAN Detox Cleanse. (2020). Retrieved from https://cancancleanse.com/how-to-lose-weight-with-a-juice-cleanse/

Marie Issels, I. (2001). Information on detoxification and the organs that remove toxins. Retrieved from https://issels.com/publication-library/information-on-detoxification/

Palermo, E. (2015). Detox Diets & Cleansing: Facts & Fallacies. Retrieved from https://www.livescience.com/34845-detox-cleansing-facts-fallacies.html

The juicing diet has similarities to the raw food diet in that it is largely based around raw fruit and vegetables. (2019). Retrieved from https://www.diabetes.co.uk/diet/juicing-diet.html

The Science Behind the Benefits of Doing a Juice Cleanse – The Juice Truck. (2019). Retrieved from https://www.thejuicetruck.ca/blogs/news/the-science-behind-the-benefits-of-doing-a-juice-cleanse

Wong, C. (2020). What Is a Juice Cleanse?. Retrieved from https://www.verywellfit.com/juice-cleanse-89120

Made in the USA
Las Vegas, NV
01 May 2021

22327538R00108